# PLEASURES

## WOMEN WRITE EROTICA

# PLEASURES

## WOMEN WRITE EROTICA

*EDITED BY*

# LONNIE BARBACH, PH.D.

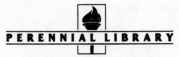

**PERENNIAL LIBRARY**

Harper & Row, Publishers
New York, Cambridge, Philadelphia, San Francisco
London, Mexico City, São Paulo, Singapore, Sydney

# CONTENTS

| | |
|---|---|
| *Acknowledgments* | viii |
| *List of Contributors* | viii |
| *Introduction* | ix |

## I

## THE RELATIONSHIP       1

### INTIMACY

| | |
|---|---|
| *Awakening* BY SUZANNE MILLER | 9 |
| *Healing* | 13 |

### FIRST EXPERIENCES

| | |
|---|---|
| *Seventeen Years, Take Note* BY LYNN SCOTT MYERS | 19 |
| *The Find* | 33 |
| *Autumn Loves* BY VALERIE KELLY | 46 |
| *Viyella* BY SUSAN GRIFFIN | 60 |
| *The Way He Captured Me* BY SHARON MAYES | 70 |
| *Malaquite* | 85 |

## II

## QUALITIES OF EROTIC MOMENTS       97

### ANTICIPATION

| | |
|---|---|
| *Sailing Away* | 109 |
| *Siblings* BY DOROTHY SCHULER | 117 |
| *Picasso* BY MARY BETH CRAIN | 122 |
| *1968* BY SIGNE HAMMER | 133 |

## PLAYFULNESS AND HUMOR

The Fifty-Minute Hour: Between the Minutes...    139
How I Spent My Summer Vacation    148
Truckin' BY BROOKE NEWMAN    164
Screaming Julians BY GRACE ZABRISKIE    168

## THE PHYSICAL

The Work to Know What Life Is BY DEENA METZGER    183
The Drainage Ditch    186

## THE CONTEXT

Tropical Places    189
The Bull Dancer BY DEENA METZGER    204

## POWER

A Few Words on Turning Thirty in Marin County,
  California BY CAROL CONN    211
And After I Submit    221

## TRANSFORMATION

Prisoners BY SYN FERGUSON    229
The Growing Season BY JACQUIE ROBB    250

## III

## THE FORBIDDEN    265

### GROUP SEX

Morning Light BY BETH TASHERY SHANNON    273
California Quartet BY HELEN A. THOMAS    285
Rub-a-Dub-Dub...    298
Evesdropping    309

## ANONYMOUS SEX

*Women Who Love Men Who Love Horses* BY SUSAN
  BLOCK                                      317
*The Moon Over SoHo*                         329
*A Very Special Dance* BY CAROL CONN         338

Biographies                                  341

# ACKNOWLEDGMENTS

As always I would like to thank my editor Loretta Barrett and my agent Rhoda Weyr for their continued support as well as Cherie Martin Franklin for her editorial assistance. Lucinda Mercer, Danny Slomoff, Bob Cantor, Joe Barber, Cherie Adrian and Robert Kutler all devoted time to reading the manuscript and provided me with important feedback.

Given the large number of authors, this project turned into an administrative nightmare. Without the help of my assistant Rosalie H. Moore, who handled all the correspondence, typing and general day-to-day details, this book might never have come into being.

Finally I would like to express my appreciation to all of the authors of the stories contained within. Their willingness to share a very personal part of themselves is truly what made this book possible.

I thank you all.

# LIST OF CONTRIBUTORS*

Carolyn Banks, Lonnie Barbach, Susan Block, Wickham Boyle, Carol Conn, Tee Corinne, Mary Beth Crain, Syn Ferguson, Susan Griffin, Signe Hammer, Robin M. Henig, Valerie Kelly, Marian Kester, Sharon Mayes, Karen McChrystal, Deena Metzger, Suzanne Miller, Lynn Scott Myers, Brooke Newman, Doraine Poretz, Jacquie Robb, Rayann St. Peter, Dorothy Schuler, Beth Tashery Shannon, Helen A. Thomas, Grace Zabriskie

*Due to concerns about privacy, some authors have chosen not to place their names on their stories. In addition, two authors preferred to remain totally anonymous, and their names do not appear on this list.

# INTRODUCTION

Since 1972 I have been working with women, to help them resolve their sexual problems. From early on in my work, I became aware of the absence of erotic material oriented expressly for women. Yet there appeared to be a tremendous need for written material that could assist women in creating an erotic frame of mind, not only to help them become orgasmic but also to increase their level of desire. The few books that were available were greatly appreciated. *My Secret Garden* and *Forbidden Flowers*, compilations of women's sexual fantasies by Nancy Friday, were recommended again and again. Anaïs Nin's books, even though written explicitly for a male patron, were among the women's favorites. *Fanny Hill: Memoirs of a Woman of Pleasure* by John Cleland and *The Pearl*, written anonymously, were also found enjoyable. But, with the exception of a scene or two in romance novels, or *Fanny* by Erica Jong, or *Blue Skies, No Candy* by Gael Greene, not much else could be found in local bookstores. Most women felt uncomfortable with the idea of patronizing sex shops and "adult" bookstores, and those who did so complained that the writing was male-oriented, that the sexuality described was not arousing to them, and that it reflected attitudes and experiences they could not identify with.

Over the next several years, the idea for a project on female erotica continued to germinate in the back of my mind. Then in 1977 I went traveling for nine months to escape the stresses and pressures of my writing and research. In the course of my travels, I suddenly realized the solution to the women's erotica dilemma. If women were to write about real experiences they found arousing, wouldn't this material by its very nature be more appealing to women than erotica written by men? Erotica based on actual experiences would also be more representative of what women really enjoy than erotica based on fantasies, which often go untested. Furthermore, since sexual images in our culture tend to be male-dominated, fantasies would be more likely to reflect a male point of view than would accounts of real experiences. Therefore, a book based on women's real experiences would not only produce useful material to help women learn to be orgasmic or to increase their level of desire, but would also document an area of female sexuality which has rarely been written about.

Even though I knew that the project was an absolute necessity, I hesitated to begin it. I, too, was affected by the cultural bias that female eroticism is somehow dirty or degrading. I was concerned about my career. I was already much younger and more unconventional in my approaches than most people in the sexuality field. I felt that my reputation and credibility were not in a position to survive the onslaught of criticism that a book like this could easily generate. So I put the idea on the back burner to await a more auspicious moment, when the culture would be more accepting and my own professional competence had become more firmly established. And finally, after years of hacking away at the subtle forces that deemed women second-class citizens in the bedroom, undeserving of sexual pleasure, inhibited and embarrassed about their bodies and sexual feelings, I finally felt the time was right.

I wanted to create a collection of women's real sexual experiences that would be arousing to women and would give them permission to feel good about their sexuality and sexual activities. And I wanted it to be written by a number of authors so that a variety of women with different attitudes and experiences could be represented. Contributions from straight women, lesbian women, married, single, conservative and liberal women could more fully describe the variety that exists in female sexuality than the experiences of one writer alone.

In documenting a range of sexual activities that women actually engage in and enjoy, I hoped to help female readers more fully accept their own sexual preferences and experiences they might have otherwise felt were unusual or unnatural. The contributors concurred, and many agreed to write stories because of this. "It's a permission giver," one writer offered. "Readers will see that, regardless of what they have done sexually, they don't have to feel ashamed." Susan Block, another contributor, stated, "I'm intrigued to read the experiences of other women to find out how they are different from or similar to my own. This book will set up better communication among women on subjects women don't publicly communicate about, and I think that is a very positive breakthrough."

After twelve years as a psychologist and sex therapist, I am convinced that women are more satisfied and self-confident when they can truly feel good about and celebrate their sexuality. An enjoyable sex life not only provides women with a multitude of physical pleasures but can add immeasurably to the stability and satisfaction of a loving emotional relationship. It is healthy for women to feel sexual, to think about being sexual, to write about their sexual feelings in the same way they write about other aspects of their lives. As one of the contributors, Wickham Boyle, said, "The reason this project excited me so much was that so often writers protect themselves behind their characters. Women are erotic. They think these things; they do them; and we should be able to write them down without being embarrassed." Clearly the other contributors agreed.

You might wonder where I found these women, women who

were willing to put on paper some of their most intimate experiences. I began first with friends. Many of my women friends are excellent writers and I asked them what they thought about the project. Their response was overwhelmingly positive, and four of them ended up submitting stories. After this, I approached other writers whose work I admired. I wrote over a hundred letters to novelists and nonfiction writers inviting them to contribute to the anthology. I was heartened that even though very few accepted, almost all responded to my inquiry, and many offered words of support and good wishes. If nothing else, I compiled an impressive file of autographs.

Writers declined to participate for many different reasons. Most either had no interest in writing erotica or were fully consumed by their own literary projects. One writer specified that while she wrote romance novels, she felt her reputation was based on *not* writing sexually explicit material. And a number of other writers, while willing to write erotic fiction, were hesitant to write about real experiences. One writer expressed reservations I myself was concerned about. She wrote, "Do you honestly think that a collection such as the one you describe will not be marketed as love secrets of famous writers or worse? It seems to me that it is not the skill of professional writers that is being sought, but rather the titillation involved in the exposure of their private lives."

To counter this concern, I offered contributors complete anonymity; there was no requirement even to place their names on the list of contributors, much less on their individual stories. However, the fact that they were to recount a real experience remained a concern to some writers. For example, a quite well known writer responded by saying, "I think it was the 'real experience' stipulation that really threw me. On thinking it over, I realized that few if any of my erotic experiences had any narrative potential whatsoever; good sex, to put it suc-

cinctly, is not necessarily a good story. Besides, I found myself
up against the wall of my own embarrassment; even the protection of a pseudonym seemed inadequate."

Some women did not want to be restricted to real experiences
because they felt they were far inferior to what they could
create in fiction. "Do you really want real experiences?" one
woman wrote. "Mine are awfully depressing, by and large.
However, I have some fictional scenes that are quite exciting."
Another said, "Alas, I am sorry to say that I cannot recall any
turn-on real-life experiences. I live a very bland existence. The
only fun I have is with my book characters."

The major reason writers opposed the real-life-experience
requirement, however, was their feeling of being straitjacketed.
One well-known author expressed it this way: "I am opposed
to the stipulation that the writing be limited to 'real personal
experiences,' both from the point of view of a fiction writer
and on the general grounds that it seems an unnecessary, and
potentially crippling, restriction on any writer. To write such
a story, the writer would, by definition, require the same freedom—to draw on both fantasy and reality, imagination and
memory—that she has in her other work." Another writer
said, "Restricting a writer to truth is like handcuffing a mime."

This demarcation between real experience and fiction intrigued me because, as a nonfiction writer, I found it far easier
to stay within the bounds of fact than to fabricate something
from imagination. Sharon Mayes had a similar experience:
"Although I usually want to fictionalize things rather than make
them real," she said, "in this story I tried to stick totally to
reality because it was more erotic in reality than it ever could
be in fiction."

At times, it is hard to know where reality leaves off and
fiction begins. Even with the best of intentions, in re-creating
an experience from memory, we remember what we want to

remember, add what is missing, and omit that which is less than desirable. In this sense, there may be no such thing as "real experience" when memory is relied upon. In addition, fantasy and reality often become thoroughly intertwined in a sexual experience. So while I understood some of the writers' objections, I nonetheless wanted to base this first compilation on encounters the women had really experienced. I felt that stories at least based on real experiences would give the anthology documentary value as well as value as erotica, and I could always expand to fiction the next time around.

Luckily, there were other women who felt the same way I did, and finally, after months of correspondence, I began to receive unsolicited inquiries based on word of mouth. Even a few writers who were unable to submit stories themselves were still enthusiastic enough about the project to enlist others. Joanna Russ was one of the women to whom I am most grateful; Judy Brown is another. And after almost one year and just under a hundred submissions, I chose thirty-one to include in this volume. The contributors, over a third of whom were married or living with a partner, ranging in age from twenty-six to forty-seven, were recruited from such states as New York, California, Oregon, Texas, Maryland, Georgia, Colorado, Kentucky and Tennessee. The authors did not specialize in writing erotica. In fact, with the exception of a few, it was their first attempt at a specifically erotic theme.

The writers come from a wide range of backgrounds and experiences. For example, one writer reported, "I've slept with only one person in my life, and I've been married to him a long time. So I wondered if anything had ever happened to me that others would find erotic. But I realized that different things are erotic to different people, that it doesn't have to be bizarre to be really exciting." Other women had a wider range of experience: "Some of my best relationships began with sex and revolved around sex," a second writer said. "It can be a delicious way of getting to know a man." But regardless of what was true of a woman's current stance, almost all the women felt that their sexuality had changed over time. The second writer continued, "Now, though, I want to get to know the man first, and the best sex is when I'm already involved. I see sex as a part of going on with something that's already established."

Women chose to write about a particular sexual experience for many different reasons. Some picked an experience that was recent and hence fresh in their memory, or one that lent itself to a short story. Other women picked a particular story because it was one of their most joyful or memorable sexual experiences. Others chose experiences because they recaptured times in the authors' lives that they wanted to preserve. The author of "The Fifty-Minute Hour: Between the Minutes" said, "As I get older, these kinds of experiences don't happen as often, especially now that I'm married. Writing about it is like having a handprint in cement. When I'm seventy I will be able to say to my grandchildren, 'See, you're not the only ones who can do such wonderful things.'"

Some authors found certain incidents were memorable because they involved the unexpected, the enchanted, or something unique or spontaneous, while others, such as Sharon Mayes, picked the ordinary on purpose. "I thought my experience would be one that other women could relate to, something that others might also find erotic. My experience was more normative than unique or unusual," she said.

Ultimately I selected the thirty-one poems and stories included in this volume because they represented a broad range of erotic experiences. And while no one is likely to find all of the stories appealing, each story was judged erotic by at least one of the people who reviewed them. Incidentally, the se-

lected submissions were read by both men and women, and,
interestingly, while women often find erotica written by men
unexciting, the men who read these stories found most of them
a turn-on. As a matter of fact, one close friend's wife mentioned
to me that she couldn't figure out why her husband had been
so amorous of late. He had been virtually pouncing on her
every night. When she discovered he was reading chapters
from *Pleasures* before bedtime, she threatened to set up a ra-
tioning system!

The themes of the stories seemed to fall into categories
similar to those Linda Levine and I generated in *Shared Intimacies*
after interviewing women about the qualities that contributed
to good sex. While each story may contain a number of themes,
a major theme tends to explain why the author chose to write
about that particular experience. Most of the stories center on
some aspect concerning the importance of the relationship with
a partner, such as love, trust, friendship. Within that, elements
such as a sense of playfulness, the power dynamics between
the two people, the sheer physical experience, the buildup of
anticipation, a unique setting or the surprise of the unexpected
played important roles. Some stories involved the forbidden—
making love to someone the woman hardly knew, to a partner
far younger or older, to two men at the same time or with
another couple present or overheard in the next room. Finally,
there were the memorable first experiences, the first time a
woman made love or the first time she made love to a partner
she became deeply involved with. Unanticipated, however,
were a couple of stories which were remembered because they
were truly transformative events and one incident which, while
being highly erotic, was not at all explicitly sexual in nature.

Because so few women ever have the opportunity to write
erotica based on real personal experiences, I wanted to find
out from the contributors what the process of writing the stories

had been like for them. As with their individual sexual episodes, the experience of putting it on paper varied from woman to woman. Most women agreed, however, that it required considerable skill to convey the erotic feelings. As one contributor said, "It was difficult to get across all of the incredible sexual sensations without making it read like cheap pornography." Signe Hammer thought, "What was most difficult was to articulate a sensual experience, to find the right words to convey something nonverbal."

Other women had difficulty for emotional rather than technical reasons. One woman had such a negative experience that she never actually finished her story. In her words, "I became so involved in reliving my experiences that I found myself becoming more and more angry with the men I was writing about and more things kept creeping into the story about what turned me off as well as what turned me on. I feel that there are plenty of men out there turning women on and suddenly I do not want to immortalize them. I don't want to print only one side of the story. So as a sensual woman and out of deep despair for what I have experienced and seen around me in this man-woman situation, I choose to remain silent."

Creating erotica, clearly, required much more than merely relating the details of the physical lovemaking. A half dozen of the contributors had difficulty writing their pieces because they had not yet fully worked through the emotional relationship with the person they were writing about. "The first draft was easy to write; I wrote it when we were together," Dorothy Schuler said. "But the rewriting was difficult because in the meantime, we had a fight and I wasn't seeing him anymore. I missed him terribly. When I did the final draft I called his answering machine ten times just to hear his voice and to help put me back in the experience of being with him again." Valerie Kelly felt similarly. "It was hard to dredge up the warm feelings that I am trying to let go of. It made me nostalgic, especially knowing that I can't have the relationship I want with that person and yet wishing for it with someone." Another woman said she cried while writing her story.

However, for a few of the women, the exercise of writing about the relationship actually helped to liberate them from it. "While writing it I felt an upheaval of emotions," Suzanne Miller offered. "I personally had to go through a lot of pain because my partner and I were separated at that time. But there was a joy in being able to express it." And Karen McChrystal added, "It was a real catharsis, an exorcism, because it helped me to finish the relationship. It was a tribute to the intensity of the relationship that the feelings could endure and come out again in a story."

The contributors who had resolved the emotional relationship with their partners found the process of writing their stories both sensual and erotic. As Rayann St. Peter said, "I enjoyed writing it and it came really easily because it is about my current relationship and the relationship is good." Another woman added, "It turned me on each and every time I proofread it." Another said, "I was surprised at what a turn-on it was to write it—a sensual/sexual thrill." And another, who wrote her story in the library, said she got so turned on she forced herself to leave before she did something she would later regret.

Two of the authors used their stories to enhance their intimate relationships. The author of "Healing" shared the pages of her story with her partner as she wrote them. "We would make love one day," she told me, "then I would write the experience up and read it aloud to her the next day as a way to turn us both on. Sharing the writing between the two of us made it even more personal." The author of "The Way He Captured Me" gave her story to her partner for his birthday. "Because he has everything, it's hard to find him the perfect present, so I gave him this story. And he loved it. He said it was the best present he ever got."

For some women it was important to create an erotic atmosphere in order to write. "I couldn't do it if I felt depressed or ill," said one contributor. "I had to be feeling good and sensuous. So it was hard to find the right moment to write because I had to be in an atmosphere that allowed for sexual feelings and thoughts."

While some women welcomed the opportunity to put forth their ribald and earthy selves, others found the process of describing sexual reality embarrassing. They talked about feeling vulnerable and exposed because the subject matter was so intimate. Carolyn Banks said, "It's hard to write about myself and not hide behind a character. I don't write confessionally, so this frightened me." Many did not feel comfortable showing their pieces to colleagues or friends. If they did share their work, they picked those they showed it to very carefully. Robin Henig related the following humorous story that illustrates the potential for embarrassment only too clearly: "I was writing my erotic story on a word processor. The repair man was there and I didn't know which disk the story was on. As he was inserting different disks I realized how embarrassed I would have been if he had seen it."

This theme of embarrassment and vulnerability affected so many of the contributors that this is probably one of the few anthologies ever compiled where over one third of the writers chose to omit their names from their stories and forgo the deserved credit. Two writers were so concerned about their affiliation with this project that they preferred that their names not even be included in the list of contributors.

Other women, however, felt they had nothing to hide and were proud to have their names associated with their story. As professional writers, they considered no subject exempt from written expression. As Syn Ferguson said, "What I write is my profession and I wouldn't do it if I felt ashamed of it." Dorothy Schuler added, "It is the literary value I'm interested in; the rest doesn't matter."

Some were proud to be part of the project because they felt they were helping other women through their work. For example, Sharon Mayes stated, "I don't find the erotic part embarrassing. I feel good about it, and I think women should share their erotic experiences. This will help other women get over some of the repression they experience in relationship to men and sex." Others, rather than feeling exposed, felt that their erotic experience was so beautiful they wanted to share it with the world.

Those women who chose to omit their names from their stories did so for reasons ranging from professional concerns to fears about reactions of family members and friends. Some contributors felt that writing erotica could hurt their reputation as a writer. "I don't think people would recognize me professionally if they knew I also wrote this stuff," one woman offered. Another was afraid she would be considered perverted and sex-obsessed if her name accompanied erotica.

However, the fear of being personally exposed was the major reason women did not want their story to be identified as theirs. For example, I was concerned that, given my standing as a psychologist and a professional in the field of sexuality, I would be criticized for being unprofessional or exhibitionistic if my name were associated with a particular sexual experience. Another therapist omitted her name because she did not want her patients to know about her personal life. Others just did not feel comfortable making their private experiences and feelings public. "It's like taking my clothes off in front of strangers and I would feel exposed in that way once the book came out," one woman said. Tee Corinne added, "I live in a rural area. I feel vulnerable about this kind of writing. It reveals a whole lot about who I am. So while I'm willing to tell people I wrote it, I don't want just anyone, publicly, to know who I am. I'm afraid that my sense of privacy would be violated."

This last reaction was the most common. The authors were not ashamed of their experiences, but they wanted to be able to pick and choose those people with whom they would share this intimate and vulnerable part of themselves. "I don't want to have to explain or justify anything about my sexual life," said one writer. "I want control over how I'm seen. I reserve that special fun sexual side of me for particular people. I don't want to share that kind of personal thing with everyone, especially not with someone who would disapprove of it. It would detract from the experience."

Some women had unique reasons for omitting their names from their stories. A few feared that readers would find their personal sexuality strange, foolish or in some way unacceptable. One woman did not want to be identified with feminist or lesbian issues. Still another woman was in the midst of a lawsuit with the man she wrote about and felt that any possible association he might make with the story could potentially hurt her case. And, half humorously, half seriously, another obeyed the wishes of her father, who, as he was being wheeled into surgery, begged her to consider the possible reaction of a future mother-in-law.

But by and large, women were more concerned about the reactions of their immediate family, their husbands, children or parents, than about those of some unknown stranger. Since concerns about mothers' reactions were the most common of all, women willing to identify themselves with their stories were either unconcerned with their mothers' response or felt supported by their mothers. As one woman said, "If it's the truth, it's too bad if my mother doesn't like it. If you are writing the best you can, why wouldn't you put your name on it?" And said another, "I don't know what my parents would think about my personal sex life, but it really doesn't matter." A few had told their mothers about the project and they seemed to approve of it. Mary Beth Crain mentioned that even though her mother's cheeks might flame when she read it, she was filled with pride that her daughter was going to be published. "However," she continued, "my mother suffers from the 'being-all-dressed-up-with-nowhere-to-go' syndrome: it will be hard for her because she won't be able to show the book to anyone because they might disapprove."

Thus I think you will find that the women who contributed to this volume are not that different from other American women. In some ways, they may be more comfortable with their sexuality since they were willing to write about their private sexual experiences and subject them to the scrutiny of others. And they are certainly much better than average writers. But they had the same concerns most other women would have about participating in a project of this nature: they just did it anyway. And while some contributors may not have written in a style that every reader will be comfortable with, I think each author, in her willingness to extend herself and expose some of the most intimate parts of her personal being, has helped to engender a cultural understanding that adventure and enjoyment in sex are positive aspects of female sexuality to be celebrated with pleasure and joy, not shrouded in guilt and discomfort. We hope you agree.

—LONNIE BARBACH

# I

# THE RELATIONSHIP

Both women and men consider the emotional relationship between the two people to be the most important quality accounting for good sex.* The caring, trust, familiarity, love and even commitment can mean the difference between a satisfying physical experience and something much more profound. When the emotional and the physical combine, there can be a kind of spiritual union, a merging, an energetic exchange that transcends the physical realm and catapults the lovemaking into something far greater.

More than half the stories in this anthology are grounded in the importance of the emotional relationship. However, I have chosen the stories "Awakening" and "Healing" to illustrate this aspect of female eroticism. While one story is about a heterosexual relationship and the other involves a lesbian relationship, both express a tenderness and connection that is rarely found in erotic writing. In these two stories, the intensity that occurs with an initial sexual experience has deepened into a profound sense of intimacy and trust.

According to Suzanne Miller, author of "Awakening," it took a period of years to develop the kind of trust in her partner that allowed her to abandon herself so completely to the instinctual experience of the lovemaking. She says, "This particular incident was the beginning of a different kind of erotic relationship, one where I was deeply touched. I experienced transcendence, the ability to go beyond myself in an erotic experience. The sex was intense, multifaceted and truly ecstatic. It involved a complete surrender to the experience of

*Lonnie Barbach and Linda Levine, *Shared Intimacies: Women's Sexual Experiences* (Garden City, N.Y.: Anchor Press/Doubleday, 1981). Linda Levine and Lonnie Barbach, *The Intimate Male: Candid Discussions About Women, Sex, and Relationships* (Garden City, N.Y.: Anchor Press/Doubleday, 1983).

3

eroticism which was very different from just two people making love together. Instead of an erotic exchange, I felt there was no longer a 'me'; there was no separation between me and my partner. The experience I wrote about was the first time this had happened, and it defined erotica for me. As a result of that experience, I was freed from my cultural conditioning about what was 'supposed' to be erotic."

"Healing" is similar in that the incredible caring and love come through in every encounter. Both the author and her lover, who have been together five years, seem to be highly sensitive to the needs of the other, sexual and otherwise. And in addition to expressing the love and tenderness shared in their relationship, there was another reason the author of "Healing" chose to write about this experience. She received the invitation to participate in this anthology shortly after undergoing surgery for a hysterectomy. "At the time," she said, "I thought that if I came through this still being sexual, I was going to write about it. My physician gave me no useful information, so I hoped that writing this story would help fill a gap for other women."

### First Experiences

A woman's first lovemaking experience often remains indelibly etched in her memory. Not that this experience is always among a woman's best, but when the emotions are right, the partner is tender and caring, this first time can be an extraordinarily wonderful experience. In "Seventeen Years, Take Note," Lynn Scott Myers re-creates her first sexual experience with a lad from the British countryside, and the feelings of pure, innocent young love are clearly expressed. Quite often, such youthful relationships end, and rarely do we get the opportunity to reencounter a first love later in life. However, after Lynn submitted the story, she returned to England to find Darrell and recapture what might have been left of that magical experience. Sadly she reported, "I am back from my pilgrimage to Wisbech, England, where I discovered Darrell still lives, with a wife who raises Labrador retrievers and with their two children. The Rising Sun Inn has been completely renovated to a fine plastic finish, and all the dart holes in the walls have been plastered over. The old farmers are gone, and most of the orchards have been cut down for the new highways. The peas I ate for lunch with my fish and chips were small and scrawny because of a dry, hot summer. However, the thrill of walking down the same lane—past the Rising Sun Inn and the camp, still intact—was magnified by seventeen years of anticipation and fantasy. I didn't try to see Darrell, nor seek out our private orchard. Some things are better left as they were. But it was reassuring somehow to know that he was still right there, and I derived a strange and unexpected comfort from that fact."

The eroticism of first-time experiences is not limited to the first time a woman has sex but can include such other sexual "firsts" as making love outdoors, making love with two or three other people or making love to a woman for the first time. The author of "The Find" recounts that her first sexual experience with another woman was "deeply satisfying." She says, "This experience was most provocative because I'm primarily heterosexual and I had never made love to a woman before. It was an expression of something I had imagined and wished for but never expected to experience. The richness of the sexual exchange had much to do with the fact that she and I shared an appreciation of the senses—something we expressed in our poetry and painting. Writing it reminded me again of how wonderful the experience had been."

Another kind of sexual experience that tends to remain memorable is the first time a woman makes love to a partner with whom she later becomes deeply and emotionally involved. When the chemistry is right, the sex can be intense, yet gentle, embodying all of the potential of this special union. Four of the authors re-created such first experiences. Valerie Kelly, author of "Autumn Loves," sums it up well in describing the particular relationship she chose to write about. "This was the most romantic relationship I've ever had. It was one of those immediate attractions that are so rare. Then the physical attraction spilled over into everything else. It was my first big love, and I've never gotten over it. I guess the first experience of an important relationship remains in your mind forever. I know this one has."

Sometimes an intense and deep emotional relationship is not based in reality. Especially in the early stages of a relationship, the person we think we love may actually be a projection of our own fantasy. And yet this projection can create an intense and powerful erotic component. In such cases, however, the fantasy projection is also often responsible for the downfall of the relationship. In "Viyella" Susan Griffin tried to hide the reality of her lover, even from herself, and continued to bask in the love of the fantasized person as long as she could. "When I ask myself why this relationship came to mind," Susan says, "no single reason presents itself. I don't like to narrow the meanings by choosing one or imposing an oversimplified idea of truth on it. In fact, this itself *is* one of the themes of the story—one I am most intensely concerned with now: a wish to avoid imposed meanings or fantasies and instead let a deeper understanding of events reach out to me. In writing this story, I began to see how my idea of who another woman was obscured my actual experience of her. In this case, both the fantasy and the betrayal of fantasy destroyed what was real, or possible, between us. And yet the meanings continue growing, and what was real remains, in a deeper sense, in-destructible."

Sharon Mayes, author of "The Way He Captured Me," writes a story with a happier ending. In fact, she and the man she wrote about were married Christmas Day nine months after she submitted her story and three years after the incident she wrote about took place. Still very much in love, Sharon has words of encouragement for those who wonder if the sexual intensity can endure as a relationship continues over time. And what she says mirrors what other women in even longer-term satisfying relationships have reported. "I remember this first experience because I knew it would develop into something very intense. And it did," she says. "Our sex life has improved dramatically over the years. It's the best sexual relationship I've ever had over a long period of time, and there is nothing unusual or wild about it. But it is consistent. It's interesting because I was a loner and I never wanted a commitment again. But now, happily married, I never want to be without him."

The feelings of the first experience of an intense relationship can be heightened when some aspect of the forbidden is added. Making love to someone of a different race or different social class, or someone much older or much younger, can enhance the erotic component. Such was the case in "Malaquite," where the author describes her first experience with a man only three years older than her son, a man she remained involved with for some time to come. According to the author, "The whole age difference really added to it. Being with a man so much younger is really something of a taboo. But the relationship was one of the best I've ever had. He was kind, considerate and sensitive as well as loving."

To find out how these women who loved and were deeply loved describe their intensely emotional and sexual relation-ships, please read on.

# INTIMACY

## Awakening

### SUZANNE MILLER

Elliot's hand comes to immediate and reassuring rest upon the small of my back, as it unfailingly does when he lies next to me as I stir into awakening. I have loved Elliot for many years, and this familiar yet ever unexpected gesture continues to move me. I sometimes ponder how a subtle unabated desire for him has remained so alive and flamelike within me; familiarity so often dulls our sensitivity to the changing beauty of those we love.

We don't sleep like spoons, rarely confront issues, have not gone to therapy, and our shared time is as sporadic and imperfect as the paradoxical creatures we ourselves are. We live together, quite simply, as animals do.

Elliot's hand knows (whether Elliot himself does or not) that I need its warmth, its current, its solidity, to live. I have lived much without it, given our penchant for separations, but it is the current of life to me, that hand on my back; it is my food, my desire, my reason. From his palm to the small of my back and out through to my belly, which rests flat on the surface of the bed, Elliot's solar glow begins its slow radiance, suffusing my heart with its warmth, flowing downward like molten lava over my Venusian mound, down farther, down the insides of my legs, stirring like lights the inner spaces below my ankles.

Perhaps he is reading, possibly unaware of this journey we have begun. It is as though his instinct is ahead of him, moving him toward me, drawing him from his solitary flight. I don't know—can we ever know another's experience directly? Still, my imagination seeks images of explanation; what is it at Elliot's deepest core that knows me? I don't ask him, I feel the current travel from him through me and out again; our molecules, heedless of our possible intent, begin their rhythmic intimate dance.

I listen to the sound of birds outside our cottage, then the sound of our breathing, now in unison, all of my senses coming alive. This time, this unique and unrepeatable time, I hear the rustling of a page. A magazine falls softly to the floor. Moments pass and his hand changes pressure slightly. Our breathing is slow, rhythmic and relaxed.

My eyes, resisting morning, are still closed and I am awake within that light-darkness. Elliot is wordlessly aware that I am awake; our ritual is silence. We are orphan-close, so far away in this moment from the day which will soon press upon us. We are farther still from our differences, our troubles, far from who we often pretend we are, even to each other.

Elliot withdraws his hand, as he turns on his side toward me. I feel a momentary emptiness, a longing, as the current subsides and begins again as he replaces his hand. Past images come at me like dreams as he moves closer. Elliot on his knees, gripping my arms as I sit, blocked from him by fear, pulling me down to meet him, his eyes calling me out from my defenses, where we can touch. I remember a San Francisco street corner and Elliot's arm encircling my waist, drawing me into him as I am about to obediently follow a green light. The light, the crowd, the sounds, stopped then, as the world has now. Elliot, sweet surprising Elliot, moving toward me panth-

erlike, unexpected, with the grace of his full presence. I have
lived without knowing if he desires me until these moments,
coming without warning, taking me from who I thought we
were; freeing me.

I open to him as his hand moves up from that sacred grove,
up the center of my spine, so slow, so unhesitating. I feel lank
morning strands of my hair being caressed into beauty, tousled
farther across the broad flushed plains of my face. We are quiet
and strange to each other, private. I feel his face close over
my hair, my ear; we are still and new. I cannot breathe enough,
and am afraid to breathe, to break this timeless solitude.

I am all liquid—no bones, no muscle, no resistance, as I
turn to him; our legs cross-stitching themselves into patterns
they know, independent of our effort. My face finds the cave
of his throat where it can hide. My breasts lose their definition,
softened against his rising and lowering chest. My hand moves
up, gently grasping the lobe of his ear, my fingers softly stroking the tender skin that knows my arousing touch; a touch
that quickly banishes any daevas that might be dancing in
Elliot's imagination.

My hand, having made its familiar connection, slides down
his chest and snakes around his slight man's curve of waist,
around farther to that plateau-like center signifying his spine's
end, his serpent's tail. My center finger circles that bony terrain, gently pressing, pulling him inextricably to me.

We are old friends and new territory, we are deep cavernous
lovers, we are celebrants of the mystery. We begin to kiss, if
such tentative brushes could be called kisses. Our lips, seem-
ingly negligent parties to our increasing heat, take their time
with casual random meetings. Our bodies cling to each other
for the promise of some ultimate home, while our mouths
impudently enact their own rituals of tasting, biting, cajoling,

inspiring deeper breaths and tender urgency.

Elliot has told me he often feels fear before our lovemaking, that he thinks he always will. It must be now that he feels that primal near-terror, now, when he is so vulnerable. I am some dark chasm he cannot enter without being lost and changed, without becoming a stranger to himself. We go toward that death together, each separate and wandering in the other; uncontrollably pulled and mastered by a need so intense it defies our most holy conventions, our deepest resistances; so humbling that it makes us completely visible, nothing can be hidden. Even our sounds no longer belong to us, but come from some ancient region we inhabited long before our learned expressions.

We are floating like phantoms, I am between what I was and what I am becoming. We cannot separate now. Our joining is a threshold where we are no longer alone in the aching way we've known. We are a movement, a pulsation, nothing else; no one, no Elliot. Something at once foreign and remembered. Some great shock and shudder of surrender. Some sound of what could be death or what could be birth. A pinnacle of aliveness from which we fall, utterly into the moment, not two, but one, only one; beloved, delivered, whole.

# Healing

## GISELLE COMMONS*

*Sarah always said orgasms felt different after her hysterectomy. That she remembered how her uterus would contract first, and now that was gone.* Home from the hospital the pain begins to recede. I walk farther every day, read science fiction books, heal. Christine walks with me, cooks my favorite meals, holds and comforts me.

One afternoon I am leaning over her where she sits in front of her typewriter at her desk. She turns sideways and touches my arm and thighs very lightly, kisses me with lips gone soft and hungry the way hers can sometimes. Her voice has gone husky, surprisingly deep, a characteristic which always betrays her excitement.

We move to the bed and she touches my arms again, my breast, slipping inside the kimono. My pelvis begins to reach for her rhythmically and I open to her, raising my leg and bracing my knee against the wall. Turning she clasps my other leg tightly between hers and trails her fingers down the tube top I am wearing to support my tummy to where my fur is just beginning to grow in again. Slowly, with one finger, she traces firm little circles in the cleft of my mons. I begin to shake and wedge my hips more firmly between her torso and the wall.

Her finger dips down lower and returns to my center all dewy and slick making larger circles around the glans this time,

*Giselle Commons is the pseudonym used by the author for her erotic writing.

chuckling, as ever, at how wet I have become. Briefly I slip
into one of my favorite fantasies. The one where we have been
making love all night, she demanding that I come over and
over in a variety of ways, manually, orally, anally, touching
and teasing me for both our pleasures on and on until I move
past thinking, past my own vibrant will and sense of direction
and simply follow her wherever she takes us.

I return to her staccato fingers tapping out the rhythm of
excitement between my legs now more intense after each visit
to the fantasy. Wonder how she can bring me to this weightless
golden yearning place over and over all these years. I want
you, I repeat inside my head, I want you, make me come. I
want you, make me come. Outside my head I hear myself
making little mewing, moaning sounds, shift my hips again,
move one arm so that both encircle her neck, pull her to me
even more.

Abruptly I know I'm going to come, can't seem to tell her,
can't even say "Don't stop," am scared to arch my back, scared
to tense my newly healing stomach muscles, come so quietly
I know she doesn't know I've come. I tell her to move her
fingers down to feel the spasms and watch her face light up
at that outward and visible sign. "Oh good, you still work,"
she says. "Were you worried I wouldn't?" I ask. "Yes," she
answers. "Me too," I say and snuggle into her neck to drift
and dream and remember.

While cuddling I have an intense desire to stretch lengthwise
and go down on her. I laugh at myself: my mobility is still
severely limited. I can't lie on my stomach even for short
periods of time. I ask her to move to the edge of the bed, let
me kneel on the floor between her legs. She looks dubious
but removes her pants and slides to the foot of the bed, making
me promise that if anything hurts I will stop immediately and
let her finish herself.

Kneeling I move carefully from side to side, forward and back, ask her to slide more into the bed so that my rib cage is comfortably supported, my lower torso unencumbered. I look down at her soft golden nest and feel again that awe that overcomes me at the sight of so much beauty blooming there.

Dipping my face close I lick my fingers and separate her folds, take in that truly heady perfume. Spreading her lips with my tongue I explore for momentary responses, places where her pleasure rises to the surface. Sliding my arms around her thighs I readjust my position and relax into meditative, flowing movements with my head, tongue nudging her clit, pushing against the hood. Her pelvis sets the tempo, comes to meet me faster now, faster.

I remind myself that I'm the one who's healing. I need not hold back for her sake. I increase the stimulation, tucking upper lip over teeth and pressing down on the shaft just north of her glans. She begins to toss from side to side. I know she's coming now, settle to a steady motion, not changing speed or direction.

Wildly she begins to peak. I hold her thighs to me tightly since I cannot follow her across the bed. She clasps my head with her soft legs, cutting off my hearing of her sounds. Relaxing some, "Enough," she says, still rising to my tongue. "Enough, I can't take any more." I climb onto the bed beside her, pulling a knitted rug across our bodies for security and warmth.

Christine starts her period. I bring her hot water bottles, tea, wine, take care of her today. Think about never having monthly pains again. No more blood on the sheets. She asks if I mind if she uses the vibrator for an orgasm to relax her, relieve the cramps. I don't mind, wiggle against her, remember times we've played with the knob-tipped wand together, finding positions where we could share the stimulation, laughing, trying to come at the same time. Now she hums and buzzes along, crests quickly and then seems to melt, her body so soft beside me. She holds me in her arms as we both enter sleep.

In the heat of the afternoon I am lying on the sofa bed wearing only the purple tube top around my hips and stomach, reading. She sits down to talk about dinner and almost casually touches me there, between my legs. I come instantly alive to her and we both grin. Almost clinically she examines my labia, touching, always touching. "We could . . . ," I say. "Mummmm . . . ," she says and climbs onto the bed, straddling my leg. I unzip her shorts and reach inside but the angle's wrong so I content myself with sliding my fingers under the bottom edge of her pants, up and down her thigh.

My passion is building quickly as she continues stroking, pulling, her eyes watching first her fingers, then my face. I imagine that I have taken some powerful drug and my body is relaxing totally, worry, tensions, pain all swept away leaving me caught in some eternal present, all my senses intensified. I squeeze her breast with one hand and pinch my own nipple with the other, delighting in the ripples of excitement this sends speeding to my cunt, speeding to her movements there.

My focus gathers, tightens and then falls away once, twice. I remind myself not to become frightened: sooner or later I will come, by her hand or my own. She keeps wetting her fingers and moving them across my inner lips in wide broad sweeps. I take short, rapid breaths, relax, hyperventilate, start to climb my green, glowing mountain once again.

Deep inside I feel the clutch of a big one coming, the sensation I thought I might have lost. I let it rise gingerly, not wanting to grab at it, letting the ingathering take its own time and path until I hear myself howling loudly, becoming pure sound: unlovely, raw, scraping my throat as it shatters around us both and I find my body again, shaking, clinging to her; very close to tears.

Later I tell her that if my response isn't really quite the same as it used to be, I can't tell the difference. She beams at me and says that Gertie, our yellow Lab, turned over and sighed deeply when I came.

I am lying on my side drifting in and out of memories/sleep. Earlier I had considered masturbating, scanned my turn-on shelf: two by Anaïs Nin, *What Lesbians Do, Histoire d'O, My Secret Garden, Shared Intimacies;* decide to wait for Christine.

She returns, crawls into bed behind me. Luxuriously I shift from my reveries to her caresses, murmurs of love. Leaning over me she defines my ear with her tongue. I make small, encouraging sounds and she moves farther into the interior, circling, twining, touching. My other ear is buried in the pillow so all sound is distanced as she reaches in. She begins to tongue my ear with rapid, fucking movements. I am squeezing my legs together, sending streaks of delight radiating up my torso, down my legs. She presses my nipple repeatedly between her fingers, intensifying the almost unbearable sensations.

I tell her I am going to touch myself and begin to do so finding my clit enlarged and throbbing, nether lips all swollen. She spreads oil on her fingers and slides one into my bottom. I feel like exploding with all the tingling, jangling everywhere in my body as she plunges her finger deep inside me, in and out, in and out. My orgasm comes rushing at me quickly, taking my outer edges first, moving in waves toward my center.

Half asleep I tell her how, before the surgery, I was so scared sex would feel different in some major way that I decided not to even think about it, much less talk about it with her. She hugs me, tells me she understands.

# FIRST EXPERIENCES

## *Seventeen Years, Take Note*

*LYNN SCOTT MYERS*

When I paint a portrait with brown eyes, I always dash some cerulean blue next to the burnt umber and sienna hues. Eyes need to swim and beckon, they are the first things sought in a portrait and a human. Darrell had eyes like this, and like a portrait, he sat for me for long moments in a locked gaze, guiding me to bliss, the kind of bliss that makes you feel like a goddess. Every brown-eyed portrait I do has Darrell's eyes. Every man I have made love to owes him for my discovery and the exposition of the soul behind the eyes and behind the cock.

Seventeen years ago when I received my first holy communion penetration, I was set free, exploding upon and into orgasms that undulated my very being. It was because I loved him, too young to separate love from sex, but old enough at eighteen to know what the hell was going on. I was made for this, I thought then, this is what I was born for, the sexual revelation of penetration and receivement. The perfect creative union. It all fell into place for me, because I was an artist reaching for the aesthetic ideal. I was blessed with the splendid fortunatissimo of an erotic, loving male and cursed to think they all could be that way. The brown-eyed creature graced me, set me up forever with rollicking desire, discovering my

lust, the energy prerequisite for inspiration, adventure, inven-
tion. I got thwacked in the summer of 1966, in England, and
became a separate force as natural and fitting as all the other
separate forces, by becoming one with another.

Wisbech is a small town three hours, by rail, north of London, close to the Wash on the east coast of England. This area
is as fertile as a sumptuous young woman. Her flat belly gently
rolls, springing with lush orchards of cherry, plum, pear and
apple trees. Gulls dive the overturned earth behind the tractors
cultivating sugar beet and strawberry fields. Honey hues of
naples yellow and ocher in the barley and wheat fields shimmer
next to the phthalocyanine-green orchards and thickets. And
peas the size of grapes explode in early July, rainy July, giving
the patchwork-quilt farms with the cream-colored row cottages
with red window boxes a green haze.

This is when I arrived in Wisbech with sixteen other American students to pick the fruit. We were the idea of the local
produce company, to haul in students from all over the world
as their version of cheap imported migrant workers. There
weren't enough hands in the small town to get its seasonal
bounty off the trees. We lived in G.I. barracks left over from
World War II that were now owned by the company. We were
an illustrative international army: Dane, German, Greek, Dutch,
African, Czech, Turk, Pakistani, French, Scandinavian and
Spanish. And because of the times, Beatle Times and Dylan
Times, there were defection, rebellion, dissension, dope, Eastern philosophy, Western psychology, language lessons, celebration, music, music and more music. It was a timeless
microcosm of ethnological and ethereal phenomena, a dormitory of life, a slice of atmosphere where everything and
nothing mattered.

The produce company had local middle management of

overseers or wickers and haulers that led us to the fields every day; who doled out ladders, chalked the designated "bushes," weighed our pick and generally detested us for being foreign, hippie, happy and probably crawling with vermin. What an intrusion we were to the ascetic inhabitants, but there was symbiotic restitution: who else would pick the throbbing fruit for a bob a basket? And we loved it; the company provided three hots and a cot for five quid a week, and an uppity middle-aged homosexual called Arthur (equally detested) who bustled about in powerless pursuit of potato peelers for kitchen duty. At the local pub, the Rising Sun Inn, we were segregated to a brawling back room much to our delight, a continuation of the microcosm. The local farmers and wickers drank warm bitters, threw darts and gossiped about the "compers" and the "queer" in the front room.

I was primed for this spree. I sucked it all in, as lush and vibrant as the land I was surrounded by. It mattered not to me that the cots crawled or the soup was powdered. Nobody complained; after a day of picking and a few hours in the pub, we fell dead in our beds, to the sound of the whispering barley field outside our door, or the drops of rain on the tin roof.

My first morning in the fields I saw the cherry trees through a fine green drizzle from the back of the lorry. Two Norwegian girls finished their folk song as we lurched to a stop. We were about thirty-five hairy, haggard, winsome pickers draped in slickers. One's sex was impossible to tell under the gear. We spilled down from the lorry onto shore, laughing, excited, ready for the attack. I stood in front of a "bush" and marveled at the cherries, so luscious and bursting the branches wept. The blatant cadmium red and alizarin crimson called to me, the viridian green leaves stuck to my cheeks as I plunged for the fruit deep within. I picked with the juices running to my armpits. I ate and sucked. My fingers turned red and raw, my lips blazed blood. I danced. I sang in the green haze. It was Christmas.

I took my first four baskets to the weigh station and got in line behind a smiling Turk. For the first time I saw, up close, the tweedy wickers, the local chaps who managed the event. Straddled on a tractor behind the weigh table I saw a young, robust fellow, the same one who had met us at the station with the lorry two days earlier, who had stunned me with his calculated stare. He was the youngest of the group of four surrounding the small wooden folding table featuring a scale and a box of tin "farm" money. They had enjoyed my what must have looked like half-witted alacrity in the wet mist. One gent, about fifty, with a flat cap, a ragged herringbone jacket with leather patches at the elbows and thick wool pants tucked in black wellingtons, sat back and dabbed his eyes. "Ye like aur bushes, do ye, mate?" The one on the tractor razed me with his quiet stare, never spoke, just grinned. He had on a knitted cap pulled askew over a tangle of brown curls, his thick hand-made sweater over a flannel shirt was pearled by the mist. Blue jeans wrapped around massive thighs were rolled on top of high leather-laced boots. Embarrassed, I shuddered to avoid his constant visual contact while I collected my money. I clumped back to my bush, burning, past a Spanish tonadilla, a Greek nomos chant and a chorus of typical American complaints.

After a glorious day, we straggled back on the lorry, wet to the bone, farm money jingling in our jeans. We collapsed under the trees that rolled above us, gears grinding. We were a pile of red and mud. Our damp wool smelled like musk, hair pasted to faces that smiled wearily. At camp we were deposited in a heap on the gravel. I was exhilarated, inexplicably, as if the cherries I had consumed had fermented into wine.

I met Darrell that night at the Rising Sun Inn. He had come into the back room with two of his mates to watch some gypsies do match tricks. The room was crowded. It buzzed and clanked, but blared with chanson, madrigal, Lied, canzonetta, and balletto and flamenco. I sat enraptured by the sounds and the scene with my friend Louise, who was a student at CCNY. She was entranced by one of the gypsies.

"Will you look at that one, he's got no front teeth," she said, nudging me. He flashed his tongue at her, while he spun coins through his tapered fingers.

"Yeah, outa sight, bizarre." I was feverish.

"Who's the one staring you down?"

"One of the, you know, in the field." There was a roomful of girls. I did not understand why he kept looking at me.

"Ah, yes. I think you're being marked." Louise chuckled deeply, her sultry chuckle. We had been inseparable since Amsterdam, the beginning of our trek. Louise was a poor Jewess working her way through a psychology degree. Bold.

"So, you think maybe he has a bet or something with his blokes?"

"Naw. Don't be overanalytical."

After an hour of tricks and whoops and jokes, Louise left with the gypsy. She said she wanted to find out about his lifestyle, but really she wanted to return to CCNY with an "unusual travel experience." I was flabbergasted by her nerve; she left with a wink. The room emptied around ten, leaving only Darrell and his mates and a few others. I could hear their conversation now, but it was almost unintelligible.

"Aye, Darry, ye ken dole neara forty kil a doy," said the first mate.

"Nay, Peta. Beena oot to King's Lynn wi' it, whin aul check, the winnie neara blown the cran' shaff," said Darrell.

"Gaa. Darr, you in King's, goo-ann, just lik the tame you slooped the crank wi' yo teeth," said the second mate, followed by guffaws.

I got up to leave with the last group back to camp. Darrell sprang up and met me at the door.

"Ken au tek you bock to comp?"

"No, thank you, I ah, it's just down the road," I stammered.

"Gawsh, stay for anoother, then." I looked down at the floor, then at his mud-sloshed boots, over the rolls of his jeans, up his legs to the large irregular stitches in his sweater and finally to his face wearing an expectant grin.

"Well, okay." A chair was pulled out for me and I joined them.

"Me noime is Darrell, but me mates call me Darry. This 'ere's Low and Peta," he said, smiling and sparkling, clearly the leader of the pack. A pale ale was pushed in front of me, Darrell leaned in to study me and waited for me to speak. His long legs were splayed, broad back bent with his elbows on the table, one large hand clasped the other, anticipating. "This is the one au was tellin' ye aboot, Low." I cleared my throat and told them who I was and where I was from.

We talked until closing time, about the camp, American bars, American cars and how I happened to be in Wisbech. And what they thought of the foreigners, and their own jobs, and who their fathers were and what kind of cars they had or wanted. Darrell performed a trick with a match and a shilling, which he fondled expertly between his fingers. We were easy in the group, with each other, bashful, but curious. I listened intently to their speech, often asking them to repeat words. I mimicked some American dialects for them in return. There was nothing suspicious or underhanded in the laughter or the

genuine concern for each other. I watched Darrell's friends
watch him, then watch me. They loved him, I could tell.
Darrell stood up at closing time and held his calloused hand
out to me, as charming as an English gentleman. Not an eye
was cast when I rose and put my hand in his.

"Au wi' tek you bock to comp now."

I was very demure and shy and went to the wrong side of
his car, a small blue four-door Vauxhall. He laughed. I looked
at his face, the high forehead, smooth and cream in the moonlight, and the rich dark eyes that were sad and pensive. He
was gallant, secure and respectable. Exceptional. He was ad-
amant that I not come with him if I was frightened, that there
was nothing to be frightened about. I sat in the seat where
the steering wheel should have been and we were off into the
night. Winding down the glinty gravel road to the camp entrance, Darrell slowed the car and turned to me. "Au won to
tauk to ye, is that all right?" I nodded, thinking he was going
to stop right there. But he drove past the entrance, with the
wind caught in my throat, to the same cherry orchard we had
picked earlier in the day. Darrell stopped the car, looked straight
ahead, lit a cigarette and started to talk. I became mesmerized
by the song of his words, slowly tuning in, recognizing the
libretto. He talked about his urges and guilt in wanting to
burst from Wisbech and discover the world. I represented one
peephole. America, Europe. His father was a farmer and he'd
have a farm of his own one day, but after, only after he traveled,
or worked or fought or whatever, someplace. He loved his
country and his "Mather and Ba" and his brothers and sisters.
Darrell was nineteen and celebrating, himself and his land. I
listened, hypnotized, and understood. His lips, beautiful, elastic. Orating, exclaiming. He confessed he couldn't discuss
these matters too freely with his settled mates. His long thick

arms waved in demonstrations of power and anxiety. He pumped me with questions about my family and my home, comparing them to his. His energy was boundless. After several hours, he fidgeted in his seat and asked me if I'd like to take a "roon" down the lane. We got out of the car and set our mark. We raced toward a moonlit bent barn. The moon was clear and bright, not a cloud was in the sky. At the end of the lane he stopped, ecstatic, assuming a mock boxer's stance with fists raised. We jumped around jabbing playfully. His hand brushed my cheek unintentionally. "Ooee, aum sorree," he said, wincing at his clumsiness, "my lass." And he threw his arms around me and lifted me high over his head. I was thrilled. A lass.

We went to the same orchard for the next three nights. Our words flew, comparing the prejudices of our societies, our shelters. What the men were supposed to do, what the women were supposed to do. Darrell's hand on the back of my neck, or waving a cigarette with his teeth clenched, eyebrows frowning. During the day I picked in a daze. The wickers knew their Darry was seeing the Yank. I stumbled merrily along with my baskets of plums now, under the secret stare of him. He wanted to see just how responsible I was with the piece of him he was giving me. By the sudden charming attention I received from the wickers, I knew he was being as responsible. I held true and protected him within me, mellowing. I was the only American left in camp now. Louise, restless, continued to Edinburgh without me.

My not going with Louise was the sign he wanted. We did not discuss our explosive delight with each other until the next evening. He realized that I was feeling safe alone. But that I stayed because I wanted to stay, capable of making my own decisions with no demands or expectations from him. He talked about the coming potato harvest, the change of season in

August with the new type of wind that would come down from the Wash. And would I like to ride the tractor with him the next day to cultivate some strawberry fields. Darrell stopped in midsentence and looked at me, then drew me to him with his arms. I looked at his face so white and pale in the evening shadows; a light rain was falling, whispering. His sad brown eyes rested on mine in a long gaze. He pressed his arm around my shoulder, I went to his lips and we surrounded each other warmly in our thick sweaters in a relieving floodwash of ecstasy. He moaned softly and released a sigh of fervent relief, breathing against my cheek, "My strong lass, my lass, my lass." I tumulted in uninterrupted splendor; the smells of him, the feel of his prickling chin, the softness of his neck, the wet of his cheeks, his strong heartbeating embrace. I kissed his eyes, I held the back of his curly head and pressed my lips to his, overcome by the sincerity of him. He kissed me, as if he were a composite of despair and anguish.

"Ye know, I moost make luv to you, my dear lass. When you are ready. I know yer vergin."

"Yes," I said without hesitation.

"Ye neveer forget the furst."

"I know." I faced him, looking directly into him, not knowing what to say, but wanting to say so much. He traced his finger down the side of my face to my lips.

"Tomorra," he said.

"Okay."

"I wont ta be the furst." We embraced and kissed until my chin was raw from his beard and my lips were numb. Happily, anticipating our "marriage," we raced again down the lane in the drizzle that evening. He let me win and came up from behind, lifting me high, twirling.

Darrell met me at the door of the Rising Sun the next night.

He wore a wool jacket over a white shirt, and a pair of slacks, no boots. He was clean-shaven and smelled of Old Spice. I wore a white sweater and a brown skirt and stockings, trying to appear inconspicuous. The camp people trooped in the back room, ignoring us. I went into the front room with Darrell, for the first time. The wickers were there and the old farmers with their noses in their dark-brown pints. Peter and Lowell waited for us at a table next to the fireplace, the mantel laden with carved wooden ducks and pewter mugs. All eyes rose, because Darrell was to them the ideal, the youth with promise, and he was presenting his lass. The Yank. A foreigner. I was chosen, so to speak, and given complete acceptance because of the position of their favorite son. They nudged each other. We sat down with his mates and the room buzzed. I was the center of attention, the blood ran thick in that room. Yes, this was the Yank, and this was the night he was going to make her his own. I hadn't realized the magnitude of it all. It was so simple, but eloquent, formal yet gentle and natural. My face was hot, Darrell was puffed up like a peacock, abashed at the attention. I was as gracious as possible, a blushing bride. There was no stopping now.

We drove to the cherry orchard, clouds rolled by the moon, turning the shadows from green gray to violet. I surrendered to Darrell's warm gaze, glad to be alone with him at last. He took me in his arms and marveled that I was his queen, I had gone before his public with eloquence.

"I luv you, my dear, dear darling," he said. "I wont to please you, so you'll neveer forget." He buried his face in my neck and put his hands under my sweater for the first time, cool, on my back, pulling me to him, sighing. I kissed him, exalted, trembling at the electricity of his touch.

"Darrell, I am overwhelmed, I—" He stopped me with a kiss

and took my hand. He led me to the back seat, opening both doors for room. He took off his jacket and put it in the front seat, then sat beside me. We whispered to each other softly; Darrell covered my face with gentle lips, as if I were a bountiful human shrine. He put his hands on my back, murmuring in my ear his desire for me, and expertly unclasped my brassiere. I gasped at the trembling rough palms traveling under my arms, along my sides and under my breasts. "My luvly, you are my lass, how I have waited for this." He pulled up my sweater and tipped me back, cupping my breasts gently, then kissing all around the nipples until I lay back on the seat moaning. "Darrell. Darrell." The moon moved behind a pearl-gray cloud. I looked up as I felt his tongue softly on my right nipple. I closed my eyes, heaving my breasts, pressing him to me. He swept his cheeks and his ears and his hair across me. He raised himself over me and kissed my open mouth. I felt the small of his back through his shirt, his shoulders, the muscles taut in his arms. Like a blind person I traveled to his chest and felt his erect nipples. He put his entire weight on me, whispering into my ear and my neck. I looked out, through the green, the glow of the moving light, pressing his curly head to my lips. My sweater was pulled up to my neck. Darrell sucked my left nipple while he pulled up my skirt. He felt my warm thighs above the stockings with his fingertips. Then kneeling on the floor he doubled over and rubbed his lips on my thighs, unhooking my stockings from the garter belt. He pushed the stockings down with his tongue then gently kissed along the edges of my panties, his wet tongue slipping under and into my pubic hair. I loved him. I ached.

The ghostlike bushes quieted to watch. The sweet smell of the wet green and the earth covered us. The moon disappeared. Darrell stood up outside and took off his shirt and undid his pants. I saw his powerful chest and biceps. I lay on the seat writhing. He washed over me, warmed me, kissing, pressing, sucking. I felt his smooth back, his armpits, hot. I pulled him to me to kiss to find his tongue with mine. I sucked his lips, his cheeks, his neck, as he pressed his erection against my thigh and put his hand in my panties. He rolled them down, gently lingering with a middle finger on my throbbing clitoris. I gasped. He moved his finger down to my saturated vaginal opening. "Oh gad, how sweet you are, yer so ready, so randy, my dear dear lass." I kissed him, I bent into him. But his kiss was slow, to calm me. The slick head of his cock slowly caressed my clitoris, over and over, then down, then up. Back and forth. I was so wet the seat was slippery beneath my moving buttocks. I thought I would scream, I felt the desire to be corrected, to be righted, placed, pinned. I squirmed for restitution, my legs spread, my back arched. "Aum going in, lass. I luv you, my strong lass," Darrell whispered, rasping, breathing hard, whispered as if to put some controls in. He kissed me very gently. His cock slid slowly and stayed at the mouth of my watering vagina. He pushed up, steering the head of his cock into my fragile membrane. He pushed in slightly, then out, then back in, each time his cock crept a little deeper. "Au don wont to hurt you, my luvly," he gasped.

"Oh, please, please, oh my god." I grabbed his shoulders, bringing up my knees, hoping to resolve, to press him through the obstacle, to get closer to him. Exquisite tremors erupted somewhere at the base of my spine. I could no longer control myself and reached for his buttocks, pulling him down and pushing up. A thickness inside gave way. "Oh, Darry, I love you, I love you," I cried. As my raging clitoris pressed into him and his penis rammed and rocked to the hilt, the walls of my vagina undulated. With the strength of mine equaled by his own, orgasm shuddered through me as he held his cock hard against me and in me. "AAAAAAAAAAAAA. Ahhhhhhhhhhh."

"Oh my gad," Darrell raled, "Jesus."

I was being resolved, in flood. Darrell let loose; his deep thrusts and turgid spills awed me. I clamped him to me, crying. The shaft of his penis pulsed again and again. I could feel this penetration, the surge, the blossom explode, and reverb. Darrell held me, our wetness binding. Our hearts pounded. I wept silent tears as he held me dearly, gasping, murmuring, "Darling, my sweet, sweet darlin' lass." I fell into a rolling swoon and drifted above the trees while Darrell's cock massaged the inside of me, tenderly. We held on to each other until our breathing quieted. He gently withdrew with a stream of warmth. He rubbed his wet cheeks against my nipples, then kissed my stomach. I was sailing, sailing with the clouds and the moon, the trees brushed me. His lips grazed in my pubic hair, kissed my clitoris, gently, gently licked the sides of my vaginal opening, still engorged. I felt his tongue explore, search, as if to heal any damage, kissing me over and over. I drifted. Darrell got up and cradled me in his arms and looked at me. He pulled me up to kiss me. I tasted my blood, and his tears, and salt, and earth, and leaves, and the sea, barley, plums, and wine.

Seventeen years ago, take note. I did a dumbass thing. I won't go into the six weeks of splendor, our tentative plans to wed, the cottage we picked out, the town's illustrious hospitality to our 'eavenly affair; how his family watched, titillated by our powerful union. The gifts. I won't harp on my over-analytical internalization bullshit that told me I would hold Darrell down, or he me, or we were too young, or wondering about my family far away, or loving-my-country crap. No.

I went back to the good old U.S.A. to go to school like I was supposed to. To take math, when I already had the moon. To learn languages and anthropological theory when I had had it in the palm of my hand. I became sophisticated and wore mascara. I had a hundred jobs. Thousands of miles, a thousand portraits, a thousand lovers. I've had my toes sucked, swung on trapezes, snorted stuff. Seventeen years later, take note, before the year is out I will stand again on the railway platform in Wisbech, England. I have my ticket. And through the green haze, I will revisit the honey hues of naples yellow and ocher in those fields. And the patchwork-quilt farms with the cream-colored row cottages with red window boxes. I cannot predict what will become of me. It should put a cap on my torment or blow it away: the agony of knowing I was a fool to have left.

# The Find

UNSIGNED

She drummed her long thin fingers on the table, drank the coffee and grimaced. Not enough sugar. She smiled, thinking of Marelia's shocked face. "It's poison," she would say, "absolute poison."

*Sugar pouring into the cup like sand onto her belly, Marelia kneeling, shaking her wet black curls in the sun, funneling the sand through her fingers onto Lara's belly.* Driving home from the beach, the day turning over, sinking into its own dreaming, they kissed—salt still in their mouths.

"Let's spend a week in the desert," Lara said. "I'll tell Martin I'm visiting my aunt in Palm Springs. She owns a gallery there, and he'll be happy to think I'm making contacts."

Marelia did not look eager. "I don't know; it might be hard for me to get away."

Martin called from upstairs. "The keys to the Volkswagen, Lara, where are they?"

She stared at the kitchen walls, red poppies on white paper danced before her. Again: "Lara, I'm late. Look for them, will you?"

Her thumb flew to her teeth, the skin already ragged; she pulled at it before she responded. "They're probably on the dresser." She got up and put more water on to boil. *Marelia might have time to go to the museum today.*

"They are not on the dresser. I told you not to let that damn maid clean off anything from my dresser! I can't find a thing after she's gone."

33

Her head ached. She pulled the elastic out of her hair and let it fall to her shoulders. It smelled of rosewater. Marelia had bought her a large bottle which she now preferred to the lemon rinse she had always used. Drawers slammed upstairs. *All right, all right, I'm coming!*

Martin Levin bounded down the stairs, jiggling the keys in his hand. He reminded Lara of a racehorse, with his graceful neck and heavy-lidded eyes which flashed even when he was silent. Energy rose from his legs and gathered in his shoulders; his whole body rang with electricity. She had fallen in love with that power, that energy, hoping through years of sleeping with him, eating with him, loving him, she could make it her own.

"Where were they?" she asked.

"On the dresser," he said, bending over and kissing her on the neck. "Just like you said." He rubbed his hands briskly and surveyed the stove. "No eggs today?"

"You didn't say you wanted eggs."

"No? Well, too bad. I was really in the mood." He took her in his arms. "I'll get a quick bite to eat downtown."

She felt as if he were punishing her by not having breakfast together. "I'm making coffee, and there are rolls in the oven."

"No, that's okay. We'll have a relaxed dinner tonight, okay? You make the famous Stroganoff, and I'll bring the champagne."

He smiled and kissed her lightly on the mouth. She had an intense urge to slap him. He had such an air of assurance about him!

After the door slammed, she wished him back, wanted him to take his hands and press them all over her face, to push his hard stomach into her shy belly. She wanted to fuse with him, making sure some fragment of him remained inside of her, so he would not forget to return. He was her connection to that outside world where people *got things done*, where actions had consequences. *The real world*, she thought, as she padded through the thick carpet. Finishing her coffee, she hoped Marelia would see her today.

She was attracted first by the eyes: a slow burning brown flecked with amber. Lara sat staring at the woman across the library table. Her skin was white, smooth as porcelain, and her hair a mass of voluptuous black tangles fastened down haphazardly with a turquoise piece of yarn. Finally Lara introduced herself, explaining that she was a painter, and that she would like to draw her. Would she consider sitting? She would pay her. The woman looked at her with astonishment and burst into a rich laugh that made the librarian pucker his mouth. No, she did not see herself as a model. First of all, she was too round and her nose too big. Weren't models the gaunt wispy types?

Lara smiled and shook her head. "Not the ones I'm interested in. They can be any shape as long as they have what you have. I've been watching you."

The eyes widened. "And what is that?" asked the woman.

Lara surprised herself by answering so directly, so forcefully: "A spirit. A darkness."

The woman closed her book and smiled. "You make me feel embarrassed. You are very flattering."

"No I'm not," responded Lara. "I'm a painter. I have good eyes." Marelia laughed and Lara asked, "What's your name?"

"Marelia."

"What are you reading?"

"Poems. Do you like poetry?"

Lara nodded. "Are you a poet?" she asked.

"I wish to be one," answered Marelia. "I wish to write poems that have what you say you saw in me. That spirit. That darkness. The Spanish call it *duende*."

She came in a white eyelet dress unbuttoned at the throat, her full breasts pressed against the thin cotton, her hair caught back in a tortoiseshell clip. With her was a book of poems and a box of dates which she munched during the ten-minute breaks. Lara did head studies, first in charcoal, then in sepia brown, and finally quick sketches in red pencil. With each drawing Lara grew dissatisfied, unable to translate what she saw—the slow burning of the woman's eyes—or what she had remembered: the dark freedom of her laugh.

After the session, Marelia showed Lara some of her favorite poems, ones written by García Lorca. She read them aloud, with great feeling, her hands shaping the air into hieroglyphs of sound. At one point she grabbed Lara's shoulders and swung her around: "Look," she said, pointing to a hummingbird, "isn't it wonderful? That's what I would like my poems to be like. Vibrating, alive. But still. All at the same time."

Lara felt a rush that frightened her. She wanted to bolt, but at the same time she wanted to be sucked in, to feel Marelia's arms enclose her. She shivered. She had never known this feeling with a woman.

Marelia reached for the iced lemonade and began flipping through drawings.

Lara quickly apologized, "They're not very good, but they'll get better once I get to know you. You will come back, won't you?"

Marelia smiled. "Of course. Why wouldn't I? You've made me much more beautiful than I am."

She jogged early in the mornings before Martin awoke. Moving at her own speed, stinging with crystalline air, she understood the beauty of her body, appreciated how her muscles synchronized, how her breath journeying down her lungs could not be taken for granted. Running was her bridge, and in these moments—forcing out the last spasm of breath—she felt hopeful, capable of anything.

Perspiring, she sat on the steps of her house and let the morning air sift through her. Her face flamed like the orange hibiscus which surrounded the porch. Martin had bought the house for the flowers—the hibiscus, azalea, oleander. For the flowers and for the large airy room they had converted into a studio for her. Martin supported her, encouraged her. She knew he loved her. Why then was she so often angry with him?

Lara lay back on the cold brick. She had not painted anything since they bought the house, anything she felt worth looking at. Her last show was over a year ago, and the criticisms still hurt. Nothing had moved her to paint. Nothing had been worth the risk. Nothing, until Marelia.

She stretched her fingers into the sunlight and imagined the space between comprised another set of fingers which fit perfectly into her own. Marelia's fingers were strong as they traced circles and arcs from her neck down her back across her buttocks and over her calves to her feet, massaging a feeling of well-being into her body. Lara remembered the first moment she saw Marelia naked. She had been setting up her easel, and when she looked around the canvas, there she was, an ocean of whiteness draped across a throw of violet pillows; black hair traced a line around each of her nipples, circled her navel and followed a path to the stiff mound of darkness around her cunt. Lara smiled and repeated the word: *cunt*. She had been told the derivation; it meant "to know, especially having to do with the magic arts...." It had a proud meaning, not the one reshaped and bastardized by men. She laughed quietly to herself, thinking that before she had seen Marelia, she couldn't have understood the power of that word.

Completely at one with her body, Marelia posed with utter confidence. Lara envied the soft folds of flesh, the full breasts—for she found her own body too bony, sharp-edged, without substance. "I could never draw the loveliness of you," she whispered to herself. But later, on the white-sheeted mattress, in the slanted light of evening, it was Marelia drawing—circles, arches, pathways across and through Lara's body. Marelia undressed her and took Lara's hand and kissed the palm and then each one of the fingers, slowly, attentively, as if she were blessing it, and then holding Lara's hand in her own, she guided her first around her small taut breasts, circling the nipples, smoothing the skin, and then on to her own fleshy ones, back to the narrowness of Lara's belly, and then again to the rippling whiteness of her own body. Back, forth; back, forth and Marelia whispering again and again: "You are so hard and tight. I love it. Like a piece of oiled machine. And your shoulders, so fragile. So brittle!" She pushed her back on the pillows and, using her tongue, Marelia began in the middle of Lara's forehead to paint a small circle, then across the eyelids (kissing one, then the other), the tongue running under the upper lip, then the lower lip, down the chin and then ever so delicately, barely touching (but touching) the neck, then one nipple, the other, sliding down the strong line of the sternum to the quivering belly, pressing her tongue into the navel, and then slowly, between the legs now, teasing the labia which sat exposed, ready, through the net of copper hairs, flicking past it with her tongue—back, forth, back, forth—gently licking, moistening the inside of the tenderest part of the thigh, and Marelia whispering over and over, "You are delicious, so delicious. . . ." And Lara was carried, balanced like a bead of water, rounded on the edge of a leaf, not knowing from one moment to the other what she would become.

"Turn over," commanded Marelia, and when she did she felt Marelia's tongue again, brushing her spine, wide wet strokes, down, down, until it reached between her buttocks and Lara's first thought was *No, no I don't want*— But the tongue was there, teasing her along the crack and then inside exploring, tickling, tasting, down toward the vagina and then up again into the asshole and the undulation which passed through Lara shook her cunt and her belly with a force which pushed its way up through her throat, and she gasped. Rolling on her back, she drew Marelia's face to her own and finding herself beyond herself, Lara began eating the full white cheeks, sucking the lips, kneading the chin with her mouth, her teeth biting the earlobes, the neck, until finally she found her face resting between Marelia's breasts. Slowly she placed her hand on Marelia's mound of hair and hesitated.

"I'm not sure what to do. I mean how to please you."

Marelia smiled and pulled her close. "Whatever you would like, I would like."

Lara's fingers moved gingerly among the stiff hairs thinking, *They are coarser than mine, stronger* . . . , and then one finger, then two, slowly entered the deep and wet hole, the cunt: wet and soft and yielding. First with light strokes and then pressing harder, she rubbed and played, her thumb and forefingers pressed together, then released, one finger now searching deeply, stroking, circling, and all the time watching Marelia's face, excited that she was in control of Marelia's pleasure.

"Am I doing it all right?" she asked.

Marelia's deep low laugh. "Oh, you're doing all right. Very right."

"Do you want to cum?"

"No, not now."

Lara began rubbing Marelia's clit. "Yes, that's good," whispered Marelia. "I want you to bring me close, yes, close."

Lara put her fingers in her mouth and gave them to Marelia to suck and then inserted them again into the soft depth, rubbing, stroking, in and out, in and out, and when she heard Marelia's breathing increase, heard her moan, she asked: "Are you sure you don't want to cum?"

"No, no . . ."

Marelia pulled Lara's hand up and kissed it and pulled her body into her own. Lara felt the folds of flesh engulf her as Marelia put both hands on her face and kissed her fully on the mouth. And then both women relaxed into each other, Marelia's legs caught around Lara's cool thighs. Lara's knee pressed against Marelia's soft cunt. After a moment, Lara felt Marelia's breath in her ear: "Next time we'll cum. We'll cum together. And I will scream. Do you scream? I would love it if you do."

It was practically evening. Marelia was putting on her stockings when Lara rolled over and caught her arm saying: "You . . . you give me myself. You make me feel whole." She was surprised and hurt when Marelia responded: "Nonsense. No one can do that for anyone else."

Lara gathered some hibiscus, stuck two in her hair and entered the house. She had made her Stroganoff, and Martin had indeed brought the champagne, as promised. She had wanted to forget herself, and after two gulps she succeeded. Giggles erupted like bubbles in a glass.

"You're adorable when you're high," he said.

"Why?"

"Because you're so . . . so uncomplicated." He kissed her neck. "Easier to get ahold of."

"It's hot," she said. "I'll open the window."

She returned and sat savoring her caramel custard, and he reached over and began playing with her breast. She teased: "So you would like a little of zee fruit with your custard, eh, monsieur?"

She suddenly desired him. It was the first time in a long while that she had felt playful. They had been married five years and too often their lovemaking seemed to be a part of a checklist of activities.

"Talk to me," she said. He was kissing her face and unbuttoning her blouse. The bed was large.

"What do you want me to say?" he asked.

Her imagination was full of colors. She often pictured herself in pastel, merging into the people around her. He pulled her into him: "I love you," he said.

She had hoped each time they made love to fall so deeply into his heart and body that when she surfaced she would experience, as one does in a dream, a perfect sense of him. But after he had made her cum and rolled over mumbling "Goodnight," she felt defeated. A familiar ache spread throughout her body like a cell dividing. Staring at his back and shoulders, she judged his inability to make her feel lovely. She thought of Marelia. The clock ticked too loudly, its face glowing in the dark.

Deciding against clearing the table, Lara raced upstairs, showered and changed into a pair of loose-fitting jeans and green work shirt. After fastening her hair back with a ribbon, she lugged the large canvas propped up in her bedroom downstairs. She had started it when she met Marelia, over two months ago. It was a self-portrait done at Marelia's request. She had spent most of the time painting the background, a mauve-colored wall angling into space which captured a re-

flection of Marelia's profile in a window. Using her palette
knife she began layering more blues upon the pink. Once her
paintings had emerged effortlessly. The teachers praised her
technique, her imagination. Everyone expected great things
from her (*Christ, it's flat, too flat...*), and within a short time most
of her artist friends were wondering why she wasn't joining
them in New York or Europe (*Needs more red, more depth...*) as
many of them were gaining an element of recognition while
she, on the other hand (*Can't get it, can't get it!*), had failed to
achieve any particular attention and was beginning to feel her
talent was a hoax. With each application of paint, she felt
herself digging in, digging in, struggling to make the connection between feeling and paint. Once Marelia—furious at her
possessiveness—lashed out at her. "You're always digging in,
wanting me to give up pieces of myself." Lara, stung and
amazed by the accusation, responded: "But isn't that what love
is?"

Completely absorbed in her work, she didn't hear Marelia,
who thrust a bouquet of iris in her face.

"Oh, you scared me!" laughed Lara as she pulled Marelia to
the couch near the window.

"Don't let me disturb you," said Marelia.

"Disturb me? You could never do that."

The women plopped down on the battered sofa, Lara's head
falling onto Marelia's lap.

"How the painting coming?" asked Marelia.

"Awful. Can't you see? I've accomplished nothing since the
last time you were here."

Lara closed her eyes, relaxing on Marelia's wide stomach.
"Kiss me," she said.

Marelia bent over, and Lara smelled the familiar tinge of

spice in Marelia's skin. Her lips were full and soft, the kiss too
quick.

"Does it take so long for you to write a poem?"

"Sometimes," answered Marelia. "But the more I try to force
it, the less it happens."

Lara looked up and ran the back of her hand across Marelia's
long neck. Suddenly, she jumped up.

"Oh, I almost forgot!" said Lara. She returned a moment
later with a loaf of date-nut bread. "Made without the poison.
Just honey. You like?"

Marelia smiled. "M . . . mm, I like. You know it's my favorite.
What's the occasion?"

"Since when does there have to be an occasion?" asked Lara.
"And anyway, baking always reminds me of you."

"Why, because I'm fat?" laughed Marelia. She suddenly embraced Lara, holding her especially tight, as if she were apologizing for something.

The telephone rang. It was Martin. He would be home late
and was leaving on a last-minute business trip to San Francisco
in the morning.

"Since Martin will be away," said Lara, "why don't you and
I take off for Palm Springs?"

Marelia stretched her arms on the back of the sofa and said
nothing.

"Well?"

"Don't pressure me!"

"Who's pressuring you? I'm just asking."

"I don't know. It depends . . . it depends on whether or not
Richard is able to get the project he's working on under way."

"Since when do your decisions depend so heavily on what
Richard does?"

Marelia bent forward, clasped her hands together and

touched her forehead. After a moment, she looked up: "Richard and I have decided to . . . to get . . . married."

Lara laughed. "Right. What else is new?"

"I'm serious."

Lara chewed her cuticle and drew blood.

"I'm forty years old," explained Marelia. "I'm tired of living alone."

"Is that a reason to marry someone?"

"One of the better reasons."

"Like hell it is!" snapped Lara.

Marelia suddenly looked as if she would slap her. "And us?" continued Lara. "Where are we in all this?"

"Nothing is changed. We still—"

"Oh, really?" cut in Lara. "How nice." She moved to the canvas and began working intently on one corner. "Does Richard know? About us, I mean."

"No."

"So, this means I won't see you."

"Of course you'll see me."

Lara swung around. "Dammit, how could you!"

Marelia pulled Lara toward her, and Lara collapsed like a fan in her arms.

"Please," Marelia whispered, "please . . . I love you, you know that, but there was never any commitment to . . . to—"

"I don't want you to go."

"I'm not going anywhere."

"Don't I make you happy?"

Marelia, stroking Lara's hair, smiled. "God, you can be selfish, you know that?"

"You said you were not in love with him!"

"I love him in a certain way. We share things."

"We share things too."

"I know. But you don't live with me. You live with Martin. And that's good. It's what you need. And I need something too."

"What, what do you need?"

"A place to write, some security. And who knows, maybe..." She stopped.

"What?"

"I don't know... maybe a child. I've always thought—"

Lara pulled away. "Are you crazy? Why would you want a child? At your age? It's dangerous, you're too—"

Marelia exploded, "Oh, Christ, shut up! You understand nothing! Nothing!"

"I understand enough! I understand I love you, and you're leaving me; that's what I understand."

Dozens of unfinished canvases, like obedient children, lined the wall. The self-portrait still on the easel. She wanted to call Marelia. To apologize. But she couldn't. Not yet.

The house reverberated quiet. The painting waited. And the day, the day would be so long.

All morning she painted (*Perhaps it was the anger...?*), all afternoon, into the half light of evening. Digging in, digging in, one color upon the other, fleshing out the hollow of her bones.

# Autumn Loves

## VALERIE KELLY

My son Michael and I were tossing pebbles and small leaves into the creek until the game bored me and I sat down on a rock to watch him instead. The dry fall leaves joined others as they floated downstream toward the ocean. The pebbles sank.

"Watch this, Mom," Michael says, just as he used to when he was a toddler. And I watch him and think about him and about how much I love him and then I drift back to thoughts of grown-up love. We're best friends, my son and I, but sometimes, even on a perfect day like today, I miss the company of a man.

It was three years ago in September when we moved to Santa Barbara so I could complete my graduate work at UCSB. Now that school is over, at least for me, we can't seem to pull ourselves away again. Santa Barbara is such a beautiful, perfect place.

When we arrived, Michael was only seven. We walked through Spanish courtyards, climbed rocks and stopped to wonder what each flower was called, all the time congratulating ourselves for choosing such a wonderful town in which to live. When Michael first saw his new school, which is located on a grassy knoll across the street from the ocean, he told me: "We used to take field trips to places like this at my old school!"

And now it's September again, the time for new beginnings. Time for us to move on. Yet something keeps me here, bound to this haven, and something locks me out.

In Santa Barbara, autumn is the finest time of year. No more milky veil of fog obstructing a piercing blue sky; the Santa Ana winds have blown it out to sea. Even from where I sit in this little forest by our apartment, amid tall eucalyptus trees bending to the gentle breezes, the aroma of honeysuckle and jasmine permeates the air, making it sweet. When the environment is so rich, it's easy to forget one's surroundings have little to do with one's ultimate happiness. A feeling of well-being must come from inside, and in my case, that's where something's missing. Although I have the gut instinct that moving away would solve my heartache.

Three years can be such a long time. I was a baby three years ago, so naïve and trusting, so willing to be misled and so ready to fall in love. Any man could have gotten through to me with little effort. For Lawrence, it took no effort at all.

He was a professor at the university, in Greek and Roman history. I'd been told he was a recognized authority in his field and had recently returned from a summer in Greece, where he'd acquired new information on some mountain villagers there.

It was an odd thing to hear so much about this man before actually meeting him. He grew so rapidly in stature that I was prepared to meet a giant of a scholar and possibly a genius. My latest bit of information included some personal data. The professor had been divorced two years before and had custody of his nine-year-old son. Considering it an omen that we had so much in common, I looked for the chance to meet.

One day the opportunity presented itself. Jeanne, a young woman from my French class who had been working on the work-study program as a research assistant for the professor, happened to be in the library struggling with a stack of books destined for his office. I helped her carry the heavy ancient volumes across the campus and up the stairs.

When Jeanne kicked open the door, all I could see of the professor was his back. He was writing something on a yellow pad, facing the window. Jeanne called him by his first name and he turned around.

"Lawrence," she said, "this is my friend from French class." He turned around in his swivel chair and riveted his icy blue eyes on mine.

As cynical as I'd become during my decade as a grown-up and my term as a single mother in the dating world, and as much as I hated to believe in love or lust at first sight, when this man turned around, smiling, with the end of his pencil in his mouth, I was immediately attracted to him.

His hair was thick and wavy, mostly black, with streaks of silver at his temples. The silver brought out flecks of gray in his cool pastel eyes. His lips were full and sensuous and his perfect white teeth were strong and straight. It could be he wasn't handsome by other women's standards, but to me it was as if I were looking into the face of my soul mate. I felt then that this was the face I would want to look into forever.

We shook hands and I gave him my name. His hand was large and brown and his grip was firm. I held on to him too long.

He spoke to Jeanne about some of the books she was unable to find and then took a telephone call. I realized I was in the way and left.

As I walked down the stairs and into the quad, I thought about this brief experience and tried to figure out what had just happened to me. This was the summer I had turned thirty, and as an "older" student, I had always related better to the instructors than to my fellow students. I'd dated teachers in my past, that wasn't a problem. He was older than I by about ten years. That was no problem either. Yet something was frightening me and I searched for the root of it in my mind.

For a long time I had locked myself away from emotional involvement. Though I'd always been a sensually oriented person, I managed to keep my sex life and my most tender feelings separate. Self-defense, I guess. Then recently, I had even blocked my body from sex. My purposeful rejection of this physical outlet as a mode of expression, as a substitute for honest affection, had left me vacant and a little lonely. Though I honestly held the belief that sex had been an obstruction in my progress toward personal and academic growth and had willingly relinquished vulnerability to it, I could feel a strong pull back in the opposite direction. My body had other plans.

I could feel stirrings between my legs and in the flesh of my breasts. Lawrence had done nothing more than look into my eyes and press his dark hand into mine and I had been aroused by him. It was a familiar and strangely welcome feeling, despite my former resolve.

Then, as if fate had a part to play, I began to see Lawrence everywhere—at faculty parties, in the History office, crossing the quad. One afternoon, when we were both in the mail room at the same moment, Lawrence offered me a trip to the cafeteria for ice cream.

As we strolled across the campus to the student center, we talked about school, the wonderful fall weather and a little about Grecian architecture. By the time we were licking melted vanilla drips off sugar cones, we were onto more personal ground.

He told me about a woman he'd been seeing, with whom he was gradually breaking up. She was a painter and had something to do with the art museum in town. Lawrence said she was a very serious person, who, at thirty-eight, had never been married or had children, nor did she want any. There had been some arguments regarding his son, Scott, and this had caused tension in an already ailing relationship.

I asked him if he ever dated his students. He said no, that technically it was against the rules of tenure. So I told him I wouldn't be taking any classes from him and he laughed. "That's a relief," he said, "for a minute there I thought I'd have to bend the rules a mite."

The ice cream was long gone, but neither of us was ready to let go of the conversation. We found ourselves walking to the outskirts of the campus and then climbing the hill which separated it from the ocean. It bowed around a lagoon, in the center of which was a small island. There are lots of stories about that island. Chumash Indians may have used it for a burial ground and there are rumors of buried treasure from the voyage of Sir Francis Drake. Cannon have been found on Goleta Beach, just yards from the college, and a sixteenth-century English anchor was hauled in from the bay.

We talked about some of this folklore as we climbed the cliff to the peak of the hill. I was grateful to get away from the clatter of the cafeteria and the steady buzz of student chatter. The closer we got to the ocean, the more the sound of the waves took over and carried all other sounds far from earshot.

The pathway led us around the crest of the cliff where wild grass and colorful flowers grew. Down below were the ocean and the surfers in slick black wet suits. Anise mixed with ocean spray made breathing a sensual delight. In the meadow farther up, wild yellow grass was speckled with golden, fuchsia and purple flowers. I felt as though we were walking through a Monet canvas.

Suddenly, a gusty wind whipped through the grasses with

a singing sound. Lawrence put his arm around my shoulder and asked me if I was cold. I was shivering, but I was not cold.

We climbed over rocks to reach the uppermost vantage point of this mesa cliff, yet as remote as we were, our place was still very close to the path. Lawrence rubbed the goosebumps on my arm. "You *are* cold," he said.

"Yes," I lied. He wrapped his arm around my waist and guided me over gopher holes. Lawrence's fingers seemed to burn through my blouse and the warmth of his body next to mine was enough to send me into trembling.

A jogger came up behind us and Lawrence pulled me to one side. The jogger never broke his stride. When I started back on the path, Lawrence stopped me by putting his hands on my shoulders. He looked down into my face.

I was afraid to raise my eyes, afraid he would see my desire and find me a lustful, wanton woman instead of the restrained lady I had trained myself to be. But he ducked a little and caught my downward gaze, teasing me. I couldn't help but smile. And then he kissed me, at first ever so lightly on my lips. And then again. I fell into this second kiss as one might lie down into a warm bubble bath.

Slowly we knelt down onto the grass and, still in a kneeling position, we held each other tightly—no longer kissing, just holding. I was still shivering.

Lawrence whispered my name as if he were in love with the sound of it. He smoothed the fabric of my blouse over my shoulder blades in long, even strokes.

Bravely, I looked up at him. I was sure his eyes matched mine. The black centers had nearly taken over the blue and he was squinting slightly from the brightness of the sun. His full lips were parted and moist at their center. I kissed the left side of his mouth softly, then the right, then the center. Gradually, I pushed my way through my own hesitation, the distraction of the setting and any prohibitions dwelling in my subconscious mind, until all I could feel was the kiss and all I could hear was our breathing.

My knees grew weak and I begged to be let down onto the grass. Lawrence helped me to the ground and laid me back. My hair spread out among fallen weeds and dandelions. My skirt was riding on my thighs. The nipples of my breasts were poking their way through my sheer bra and cotton blouse.

Lawrence still lingered in his kneeling position, looking down at me with blue fire in his eyes. His body was backlit by the yellow sky and I could barely make out the details of his features. He was struggling with something in his pants. I could see now that it was his erection. Long and thick, it showed through his chino slacks. He pushed it down, but it bucked up again. Just watching this gave me a rush. I wanted to reach out and take hold of the thing myself, but I didn't yet have the nerve.

Now he lowered himself on top of me, his body between my legs, and he pushed his face into my neck. I could smell the sweet scent of his skin mixed with aftershave, sweat and passion. He kissed me behind my ear, under my jaw, and in the well where my neck met my shoulder. Between my legs I could feel the rough cloth of his pants. I lifted one leg to push my pelvis in the direction of his swollen cock.

Another jogger passed by and we froze still, almost holding our breath. The runner never looked our way, but it still made Lawrence nervous. He had much more to lose than I if we got caught.

And yet with all the danger and lack of propriety, I think I might have gone ahead and fucked him right out there on the cliff. Something about the heat of the moment makes one forget what's being risked. Besides, at the time, I didn't think anything so magical would ever happen to me again.

With his sleepy eyes gazing into my face, Lawrence slipped his hand into my blouse and cupped my breast. He squeezed it gently. I could tell he was pleased with the feel of it. A rush of heat flooded his neck and cheeks. After a little fumbling, my breast was free from its restrictions and naked to the sun. Lawrence bent down and circled the nipple with his tongue. Then he sucked it. It was as if he were sucking a long nerve ending, the body of which extended through my breast and my torso, and went all the way down into my cunt, where it tugged on sexual muscles there. All I could think of was how much I wanted to fuck this man.

My hips were pressing up into his of their own volition. My breasts were growing harder and the nipples stiffer. I found myself scratching my thighs with the seams of his pants, and rubbing my clit through layers of cloth against what might have been his cock.

We must have looked strange to the joggers—like high school kids—the way we were dry-fucking with all our clothes on. Eventually, it became clear to both of us that we would have to make other arrangements.

"Where are you going after this?" he asked me, almost in a whisper.

"Home to make dinner for my kid."

"Could I meet you later?"

Did he have to ask? I told him I could see him about seven-thirty.

He calculated things and said he'd pick me up around then. He mentioned he had to watch a television program at nine on Gothic art. I don't know why he brought that up unless it was to let me know he thought we'd be done by then.

It still remained for us to get up and walk away from our spot on the cliff. I managed to tuck my breasts in somehow, though they didn't seem to fit as well as before, and I straightened my skirt, but Lawrence had a more difficult time with his cock. It wouldn't stay down. Finally he hid it behind his zipper. It was fun to watch him struggling with it, but more than that, it was really a turn-on. If it was as hard and as huge as it appeared, I would be in for an exciting evening.

I made a hamburger for Michael. I couldn't eat anything myself. Then I took a long, hot bubble bath. When I smoothed the creamy lather over my swollen breasts and pubic area, I felt the hardness of my clit. It had been over an hour by then since our cliff episode, yet my hard-on prevailed. I didn't want to masturbate though. Lawrence had earned it; let him have it.

I curled my hair and put on a smocklike dress which could be easily and quickly removed. When Lawrence picked me up, he smiled nervously, and when he touched my arm to guide me into his car, I saw that look of lust cross his face again.

Even though Lawrence lived only a mile from my apartment, it seemed to take an eternity to get there. Nothing we talked about made much sense to me. When I closed my eyes in an attempt to relax my nerves, all I could see was that hard cock fighting to get out of his pants.

At his place, Lawrence fixed me a drink which I knew I'd never finish and led me into his living room. It had a very high ceiling and to one side was a loft which served as the bedroom.

He mentioned that his son was staying over with a friend and we strained to make conversation. It didn't take long before our bodies took over and communicated for us.

Lawrence found his way inside my shift by untying it at the waist, leaving me in frontal nudity. I draped myself across his clothed body on the couch, feeling slightly decadent. We each seemed to be stretching things out, biding time and hoping we could last. My cunt felt as if it had come open at the seams, searching for cock. My nipples were erect and I was beginning to get a stomachache, which is what happens to me if I get too excited without climaxing.

Before we knew it, it was nine o'clock—time for the mandatory television program. The TV was upstairs in the loft.

When we lay down on the bed, Lawrence finally removed his clothes and I saw his erection for the first time. It was incredibly beautiful, bobbing out in front of him like a sword. His foreskin had been pushed back because the knob had grown so large. It made him irresistible.

I no longer wished to keep myself under control. I reached out and encircled his cock with one hand, pulling the foreskin down the shaft and exposing the full head of his cock, a shiny, deep-red knob already glistening with pre-cum.

Lawrence shuddered but moved closer to me. I took the tip of him into my mouth and felt its heat on my tongue. Lingering on the tender underside with my lips, I took his balls in my other hand and scraped them gently with my fingernails. Lawrence was moaning. His eyes were closed. The television cast colored lights on our naked bodies and spoke to an inattentive audience.

When we finally fell down onto the bed, Lawrence put his head between my legs and cupped my clit with his lips, then used his long pointed tongue to lick my pussy. His hair was tickling my thighs, his fingers digging into my flesh. I watched him for a while, waiting for him to stop as other men had. But he didn't stop. He clearly loved what he was doing. He was even making humming sounds like one who's enjoying a good meal.

So I laid my head back into the pillow and slowly began to let myself relax. The more I relaxed and released my body's tensions, the better what he was doing to me felt. Soon all of my attention was centered down there, on my pussy and his mouth. I became aware of an orgasm rising within my body. It was rare for me to climax from cunnilingus, and yet I knew even then that this man could be the one to do it.

He stopped, but only for a moment. He stopped to say, "You have the sweetest pussy. I could eat you forever." Then he went back to his licking. His words turned me on almost as much as his actions and I was on my way. My hips lurched up and grabbed for that orgasm.

My legs were trembling and I had to struggle to keep them from closing down on Lawrence's head. My belly and neck became extremely hot. My nipples hardened into pebbles and involuntary gasps escaped from my throat.

Lawrence inserted one finger into my cunt and my inner muscles grabbed hold of it like a vise, as if trying to squeeze fluid from his fingertip. I bent my head into the pillow to wipe off some of the sweat. And all the while, he kept talking to me.

"You're so beautiful. You look magnificent, the way you move . . ."

When the shuddering finally ceased, Lawrence came up toward me and gently inserted his penis into my vagina. He did it so slowly I could feel the folds of my inner skin scrape past the ridge of his cock. He felt big inside of me and when he was fully to the top, he touched me on all sides of my cunt. He filled me.

Lawrence was a strong man. I could see his muscles flexing

even in the half-light of the television. When he lifted my pelvis up in the air to meet his, the biceps of each arm exploded under his sweating skin. His shoulders and chest were gleaming.

But it wasn't only his chest I was looking at. His face turned me on too. If I had had a mental image of what the perfect man for me would look like, Lawrence would have fitted it perfectly. His eyes were large with thick lashes. The blue was paler than the sky, in sharp contrast with his dark, tanned skin. His hair was thick and curly and his mouth full and sensuous.

Each time I was sure we were through, Lawrence started up again. He turned me over and pulled me up doggy fashion and fucked me from behind. I thought I would never like this position, but he made it feel good. He stuffed a pillow underneath my belly and tilted me in such a way that nothing hurt. I came this way too and when I finished, he moved me again, this time to the edge of the bed.

My legs fell over the side and Lawrence knelt on a pillow on the floor. He could fuck me this way without either of us having to exert much energy. He began to insert himself in very rapid strokes. I was starting to wonder if he would ever come at all. And I came again.

Then we were on the bed and I was on top of him. He seemed to be resting, so I took over. I was straddling him, my knees bent on either side of his torso, his hands up on my breasts. I began a vibrating, gyrating motion with my pelvis that forced my clit down to the floor to rub against the base of his shaft. It forced the cock to move from front to back inside of me. I can come very easily this way and when I did, I fell onto his body almost with a splash, we were so wet.

The last position was the same as the first, with him on top of me. My clit hovered on the brink of orgasm constantly, giving in to it now and then. I was amazed at how long he could fuck without coming, and yet I was also feeling somewhat fatigued. It was just about then that it happened. I felt his body grow rigid. He was moaning loudly into my neck. I resisted the impulse to push myself up into him and suck out his cum. With breath held, I remained perfectly still.

I felt him coming into me. His fluid spurted out with such intensity I could imagine it splashing off the rear wall of my cunt. One, two, three times it came out. And then, after a moment or two, more came. Lawrence's butt reared forward with each thrust. My hands rode his ass cheeks.

He fell back onto the bed beside me, breathing very hard. Both of us looked toward the television set at the same time, attracted by a loud announcer. Then the credits rolled by. We had made love for a full hour and missed the entire documentary.

"I'm sorry," I said, smiling.

"I'm not," he said, and he took my hand and kissed it. "So when can we do this again?" he asked.

"Not now, that's for sure!" I said, in mock exasperation. And we both laughed.

As it turned out, Lawrence and I made love more times together than I ever have with any other man. We went out every night until we moved in together, where we made love nearly every day for two years.

We made love in all the usual places and a few quite extraordinary ones; in the shower, on the beach, in his office at the college, in the car. Our time together was filled with emotion, sometimes tenderness, sometimes pain. We had deep discussions about the meaning of our lives and whether or not to go on as a team. Ultimately, it was not a thing that was so easily controlled. The end came about as abruptly and unexpectedly as the beginning and left us each in shock, I think. At first it was I who wanted to be alone again and then it was he and then the affair just dissolved. It fell through the gap between us.

It's been a few months now since we split up. Michael and I have a new apartment and he still sees Scott on occasion. We're happy in our own way. There's something to be said for being involved in a loving relationship, as a couple, and there are also benefits to being alone. I'm sure if I sit here on this rock long enough, it'll come to me what they are.

"Hey, Mom," Michael calls out, his corduroy pants wet to the knees. I'm irritated to have my reverie interrupted.

"What!" I shout back.

"I love you," he says. And he throws another pebble into the stream.

# Viyella

## SUSAN GRIFFIN

An erotic story. For one thing I am in a rage at my lover. And for another my neck muscles are in a spasm so painful that moving in any direction frightens me. And making love requires movement. But this of course is a metaphor. I am going through profound changes in my soul. I know this. I can describe them to you on a minute level. But I won't. Not here or now. Suffice it to say that my muscles are in spasm because I am terrified of the changes taking place inside me. And in this state of mind I sit down to write a story about Eros.

I am writing this in a conversational style. In the language of the female realm of experience. Kitchen-table talk. This is the only way I can enter the erotic honestly. I have spent years trying to be what I thought I should be. This seems to be the only sentence I can begin with, as I try to speak of erotic feeling. Now, finally, at the age of forty, I know that I am a lesbian. This does not mean that I have no sexual feeling for men. But rather that my most profound longings and desires, for intimacy, to know, to touch and be inside the body and soul of another, becoming and separating from, devouring and being devoured, that wild, large, amazing, frightening territory of lovemaking, belongs for me not with men, but with women.

What is the story? The erotic story. The story will have to be a story about two women making love. It will have to take place sometime in a woman's life after she has been married and had a child and ended that marriage, and realized that for whatever other reasons her marriage failed, it also failed because her real passion and her deepest feelings of love did not belong to men. Which is to say it will have to take place after a certain change has transformed a woman's soul. After she has decided that she will stop trying to be what others have said she should be. After she has decided to stop lying about who she really is.

Which is, by the way, part of the problem with my neck. But I am not going to tell you about my present difficulty. It is part of my private life, which is to say it is delicate and vulnerable and does not yet belong on a page nor to the eyes of strangers. And at any rate, I have made my mind so tired by going over and over again the terrain of the present, I am aching with it, aching with rage and love. I want to reach back into the past. And I want to change that past. Not lie about it. But re-create it in a slightly different medium of fact and circumstance than that in which it actually occurred.

And why? The first reason is complex, the second simple. The first reason arises out of my knowledge of the imagination and our relationship to the past. I know that depending on who we are at the moment, we reshape the past into new meanings. And the second reason, the simple one? I do not want to reveal the private life of another woman, one who once trusted me, and whom I once loved, and still do, in another part of my soul, always will, love.

I will call her Viyella. The name appeals to me. It is not of course her real name. But I like it so that I have carried it around with me for weeks. This name has made me fall in love with this character. I am at this moment entering a real love affair with her, Viyella. This name is not anything like the name of my real lover, from the past. But she could have been named Viyella. And now the name is part of the character I create who resembles someone I actually did love, make love with, hold in my arms. This woman whom I create took the name for herself, and this is part of her character. She has a sense of drama, she and the real woman she takes after. She likes to invent a persona. She has airs.

When I knew her (the real woman or Viyella? Does it matter any longer?) she had a Southern accent. This was not put on. This was the realest part of her. She was from a small rural town in Georgia where the soil is red, and I loved to hear her talk about it and her family in those soft Southern tones that seemed warm and red like the earth itself. But she had been to the Sorbonne. The way she put it, she had upped and left all that Sorbonne shit—this is the way Viyella talked—because, honey, it was the phoniest thing in the world she'd ever met up with, it just wasn't her, she was ready to go back with the real folk, the kind she grew up with. Well, not exactly, because she was now living in Berkeley, California. She wore flannel shirts. And soft blue jeans. And her hair flowed around her head like wildlands. Her face had a kindness and a plainness, not the plainness of lack of beauty, but that American plainness which made you think of old farmhouses, the wood cut simply and then left to be shaped by the weather. Everything about her was very soft, and I feel a softness inside me even now as I remember the way she looked. Something essential about her, in the way she sat and gestured, was womanly, though she had a cocky boy's walk, and hunched her shoulders, as if her frail body were ready for a fight, and she wore boys' tennis shoes. She was a photographer, who worked as a volunteer on a women's newspaper. She collected food stamps and welfare. Did things basic (she would say), had no need for fancy stuff. But she wanted you to know she had seen better and rejected it.

Stories about Paris and the Sorbonne glittered in her normal conversation the way gold or silver mixed in eye shadow shines from a woman's eyelids. She mixed French phrases in her talk. A lovely French really. Not mispronounced so much as touched

ever so lovingly by Georgia. *Ça va?* meaning, *Okay?* got drawn
out a little longer so that one heard Saaah vaah? It was nice.
She had been there, she said, to study French literature. She
had memorized quotations from Baudelaire and would toss off
a line or two at certain moments. She had been working on
her doctorate, the story went. Only Paris became more interesting to her than school. She wanted to build a life like
the one she had in Paris again, only in Berkeley, and therefore
she spent an inordinate amount of time at cafés, drinking
coffee, which was not good for her, since she had problems
with her heart. She decided to leave the Sorbonne, she said,
because she did not want to be a dry academic. She wanted
adventure. She wanted more of life. And anyway, she needed
to go back to her roots, to see again the real people of this
earth. And this is why she returned to her own country. This
and the fact that she had to face the truth that the woman she
had fallen in love with in Paris would never be anyone's lover,
really.

But there was another side to Viyella. Another part of the
picture she painted of herself. She talked about how she loved
her MaMa and her MaMa never quite loved her back. That
took my breath away when she talked like that. A woman
sitting there, saying right out in that Southern accent, flecked
so glamorously with a bit of French, how she wanted mother
love, and how she felt rejected, how she never got enough of
that love, and still wanted it. Wanted it still. I didn't say to
myself, here is an honest person. Here is a person of great
strength, someone who can look into her soul and see her own
forbidden desires. Someone who can admit to her vulnerability,
her tenderness, her childlikeness. I did not say this to myself.
Nor did I say that I was so pleased that she had been a scholar
before she gave scholarship up. That she had proved to herself
and the world that she could be someone. Someone recognized

by European professors as being brilliant. Someone certified in the world as accomplished. Someone who spoke French, after all, who knew things. Who could dazzle and impress and then say with a shrug, "None of that shit really matters, does it?"

I did not say any of that to myself, nor other things, things I knew, really all along, about who Viyella really was. I had doubts and worries. The first time I saw Viyella she seemed at the end of her rope. I felt she was desperate and lost and looking for someone to fix her. But I forgot this first impression, or rather hid my memory of it from myself. I silenced my own doubts, and in that silence, I fell in love.

I was lavish. I brought her flowers. Sent her beautiful letters. Dressed in my best clothes and introduced her to special places to eat. I would kiss her and hold her hand in public and she admired my outrageousness. I had held back my love for women for so long that once I broke free from this taboo, there was no stopping me. I did not care what strangers on the street thought. I even imagined they liked the sight of one woman in love with another woman and kissing her on the mouth, pressing her body into the other woman's body, so that the softness of their breasts made one fine softness you might sink all the way into like heaven. I even imagined this soft feeling leaked out into the atmosphere and made people around us as happy as we were.

We became lovers. She pretended, as women are trained to do, to be not entirely available. When I called to ask her out she paused to look at her calendar, and said no first, and then, reconsidering and juggling, said yes. This increased my sense of panic. When she did not leap to say yes, I felt as if I had become the condemned, as if I were doomed to be forever turned away by those to whom I express love. This was an agony, very old. Someone I loved did not love me. I was the mirror image then of Viyella in her description of herself, a child who loved her mother and was not loved back, rejected.

But finally, finally. We went out. Kissed. And then one night we were in my bedroom together. And together we took off our own and each other's clothes, playfully, with some embarrassment, and swiftness. We seemed like boys trying to unfasten their first brassieres and laughed at ourselves. But we were not boys, we were women who knew far more than boys and hiding what we knew. Yet whatever we allowed ourselves to know then, what happened first was that a kind of miracle took place just between the surfaces of our two naked skins before they even touched. A kind of radiance happened in the tiny almost invisible place between our bodies. And when we touched, my arms around her, our unclothed breasts against each other (we were the same height), her belly against mine (the same weight) and pressing lightly, that agony in me that I felt when I was not sure she loved me became an open valley in me, a hollow weeping, a cry of such longing that had you heard it as a song you would never be able to erase it from your memory. And the valley filled with all the pain of loneliness I ever felt going back to what age? So young. So young. But now the pain was good. It was the feeling of a body expecting to be touched, to be moved into even deeper feeling. It was desire, and known in that moment also by her body, and so growing in intensity, as the desire echoed from my body to her body. Her body. Its skin, that soft flesh meeting mine took right up into it all that I was, all that I knew and tried to hide from myself, or kept secret, and all that her body knew in me was blessed. While at the same time, my body felt all she had ever felt, and wept for what she had suffered. I was led in my soul to an infinite tenderness for her. I wanted her. Wanted to reach inside her, even as I ached to have her put her hands, her mouth, in me. I reached with my hand. I

touched her. I can't really tell you because I can't quite remember, can't quite imagine anything of that moment now,
except that I had finally reached into her lips, into the red
canal between her soft thighs which surrounded and met my
hand as it went there. And I was astonished. Because she was
so open. It was so easy to enter. And I was frightened to
discover no resistance but only willingness. I was not used to
this. It was as if every wish I had ever wished had come true.
As if the world had turned upside down and I no longer understood gravity. And then she said to me sweetly and calmly in
that same Georgian voice how she was not always so open.
But that was how she felt now. And since we were standing
there, she said, perhaps we had better get into the sheets, into
the bed, perhaps this would be better. So we did, and we made
love. She put her mouth to me, her hands to me, her self to
me. I reached into and around her and sank into someplace
with her, and there was such a degree of wanting that we both
cried out and then that ecstasy which happens inside a woman's
body happened to the two of us, not at the same time, but
one time after another, and then again, as waves, up the length
of the body, and then the heat, and the heaviness, and the
scent, and then the looseness as if still another layer of clothing
had been removed, as if we had come finally into a world
which had for a moment frightened us, and now caressed us,
we were so glad, as if now we were unafraid of all we had ever
feared, and laughing.

Because of that night, and many others that followed, and
days, and time spent just sitting together, near each other, in
an ease of bliss, or glancing into the face that held that bliss,
the memory and the promise, there was something in this love
that was right. Despite the pain that came after. Despite it all.
For it, like the joy, was considerable.

In the beginning, as is so when one is in love, life was like paradise. With Viyella, everything seemed more beautiful. All that was fraught with complexity or tension seemed simple now. I loved everyone more. One evening we stood out in the cold night to watch an exquisite sunset. I could not bear to go inside for even a moment to fetch a jacket. Viyella shielded me with her arms. I imagined we were angels.

But here is the irony! We were on earth. I caught cold. And now Viyella was elaborate with her plans for caring. She was going to stay with me. Order my house. Answer the telephone. Make me breakfast, lunch and dinner. But like her plans to put on a show of her photographs, very little of this came true. She would say, "I'll come to make you dinner." And at first I was surprised when she came by, looking sheepish, or worse, pretending not to remember her promise, at eleven at night. I began to expect failure from her. And at the moment of this failure I felt, like a tidal pull, her wish that I comfort her for having failed. This was a pattern. A scenario which would have to be played out many times and with no ultimate end in sight. But though I knew this, I pretended to myself that I did not know. I lied to myself, so that I could go on being with Viyella and her failed promises.

But finally there was another promise more essential to our union which I could not ignore when it was broken. Viyella failed to be the person I had convinced myself that she was. I told myself that I found this out by accident. But really I had for a long while had suspicions, and thus I made a plan to catch her in a lie. Instead of asking her openly, "Viyella, are you really a scholar of French literature?" I plotted. Pretending only the wish to share with her a phrase from French literature. I said one day, *"Mais où sont les neiges d'antan?"* She responded as I feared she would. She knew neither how to translate this line nor where it came from. I saw a look of panic pass over her face which told me everything and she in turn saw a look of dismay and betrayal pass over my face. "Where are the snows of yesteryear?" I translated the line for her, explaining to her that it was one of the most famous lines in French poetry. She left me sadly, pretending that she had known this all along. And though I could see her sorrow, all I could feel was anger, that she was lying to me even now.

Who was she really then? I didn't ask. There were a few days of separation. She came back to me more honest. All her life, she said, she had exaggerated the truth. She wanted to be a scholar, this part was true. And she was, for a week, *at* the Sorbonne, and if she was not really a student, still she had sat in lecture halls, straining to translate. I only knew that I had lost the woman I had fallen in love with—the one who so gallantly gave up academic success for a world of real people.

I tried to love her still, but I did not succeed. Though my body went on loving her. At the thought of leaving her a grief came into my heart which was as palpable as physical pain. Despite the fact that I withdrew from her, a radiance still existed between us, a joy and even a healing, inside skin and bones, this feeling we call tenderness.

Finally weeping, even sobbing, I left her. I told her that what was between us was now finished for me. At first she pretended not to care, just as, in the beginning, she had pretended to be too busy to see me. But in a few hours, she was at my door pleading to talk it over again. I would not see her. I was afraid to see her. Afraid my body might go back to her and make my mind try to live with the deception that had been making me wake with dread every morning.

After nine months I discovered that Viyella had lied to me. But it was years before I knew that I had lied to myself. I knew from the beginning that what she told me could not be true. In the first moment I met her I knew I encountered a different Viyella. I lied to myself about what I knew and even asked her, I believe, in that unspoken way that we make demands on each other, to tell me the lies she told about herself. I wanted her to weave a fantasy for me of someone I could admire. I never told myself that just as she needed to impress me with her fantasies, I needed to impress the world with a fantasy lover. And in the same way, I did not own what in myself was lost, like Viyella, buried and broken.

This tale is a story both true and not true. It did happen in the past, not just once but many times over, not only with Viyella but with others too. And it happened before I ever met Viyella or imagined her. Many, many years ago someone I loved was not who I wished her to be. She had wanted to be for me what she could not be. She made promises to me she could not keep. To comfort myself, I wove a fantasy of her, out of her illusions and mine. She was my mother but could not mother me. All her promises failed. In my child's mind I knew this, but I could not bear the despair of this knowledge. For me, the habit of lying to myself was an old one.

"Viyella," I wrote her, a few weeks after we separated, "we can never get back together again. I don't even know who you are." And I was right. But now, after the passage of time, I would add another line: "The truth has many faces." I did know Viyella and love her in my body and I can never forget this love. I do not wish to forget it. Her openness when I reached into her and how that openness changed the shape of the world for me. There is no way to love without being changed. There is no way to write about love without changing the shape of your mind and your heart. You, sitting across the table from me, can see this in my face now. If I was feeling a rage at my lover, this has become grief. Yet even grief has a different dimension now. Can you feel it?

# The Way He Captured Me

## SHARON MAYES

I was always lying in bed when he came upstairs. He undressed fast, casually tossing his clothes on the floor. This was my favorite time of the day. He invariably walked around the room in his gorgeous natural state for a few minutes before climbing into bed. My visual enjoyment of his naked body bordered on the sinful. How can I describe him? His brown skin was like wrapping on an explosive package. He was small, but not thin, his tummy protruded slightly, his shoulders were broad, a line of soft dark hair went down his belly to his genitals. Round, that's it, and powerful, his arms and legs were powerful, but not overdeveloped. The roundness of his bottom, the firm sensual mounds of muscle that moved as he bounced around the room, sent flashes of pleasure through me. My body responded automatically to the sight of him. Sometimes I asked him to stand there naked so I could look at him for a long time. He smiled at me, anything to please you, his eyes said. My desire to pet his tummy made his getting into bed almost as much fun as looking at him. I loved to watch his cock, meaty and hungry like a bird in its nest, dripping with semen, incredibly sensitive. We had slept wrapped like a tangled vine for two years. I'm embarrassed to admit we have lived together since the night we met. Why him? Why his brown curly hair and chipmunk cheeks? Why his musky male smell and his sparkling eyes? I think it was his beautiful smile that started the entire affair.

It was December and eighty degrees when I arrived in San

Diego. The breeze was cool, yet sweat prickled on my face.
I was scared, anxious, already homesick for the man I left
behind, the big Eastern city that had been my home. Leaving
home had two sides: adventure and dread. Memories plagued
the long trip, forcing me to discover the real reasons behind
my decision to leave. It was not so simple as accepting a new
job. I was afraid of love. Anthony was the first man I had
trusted in ten years; before that I didn't know any better and
trusted them all. And more than that I had desired him with
an unremitting passion. Through the wheat fields, over the
plains, across the desert, I told myself he was too young, too
idealistic, too incapable of despising me. Then my memory
ruthlessly reminded me of the magical bond between us, that
tie that held me to him in spite of my fear. I tried to rip it
from my thoughts, sledgehammer it with rationalizations, make
it invisible with fatigue, but it remained. I remembered our
lovemaking, how he would enter me and be still for a brief
moment, then wildly lose all control and come within seconds.
My body went equally wild. The moment I sensed his abandon,
I came instantly, automatically, with none of the preliminaries
or necessities of endurance. His passion for me was raw, un-
tamed. It paved the way for my body to safely embrace him
and burst into warm, shooting rays of light, sunlight, starlight.
Making love to him had been effortless, certain pleasure, lux-
urious orgasms, as many as I ever wanted. Stop thinking about
it, stop this instant, I screamed at myself out loud. My decision
to leave had hurt him, my hurt swelled to hostility. I wanted
him to stay inside me longer, to please me mechanically. The
passion faded into a fetish for replication, the joy was lost.
My fear of loving him so thoroughly had destroyed it. To leave
him, I thought, was a crime against humanity, and I was a
criminal. I couldn't love just one man. Anthony had almost

taught me how, but only almost.

I pulled up in front of a small white house. My friend Katrina was standing in a small patch of garden pulling up weeds. We embraced after five years of letter-writing. She welcomed me with fresh ground coffee and oranges. We sat on the sofa by the front window, the sun bathing me in warmth. I wanted to be cheerful, happy to see her, but my mood was stubborn. She could see my depression and I found myself in tears on her shoulder. "You did what you had to," she comforted me. "California may change all that. It's a different world. It can open you up if you let it." I listened with skepticism. She was being kind, I thought. The phone rang and Katrina's voice lilted as if a lover were on the other end. From her side of the conversation I gathered that she was planning a dinner party for me. Suddenly, I wanted to run to my car and head for home. Adventure, I repeated to myself, adventure, excitement, something new, that's what you wanted, now try to experience it. I wondered about the man on the other end of the phone. Was he her lover? Immediately, my merciless mind took me back to Anthony.

She returned and sat beside me. "That was Dr. Dan, he's coming to dinner too. I think you'll like him."

"What kind of doctor is he?" I was disinterested.

"An adorable one, a medical doctor, a very unusual one. He's like an original California hippie politico-turned-scientist, one of the most intelligent men I know. You'll see." She sounded almost too cheery, and my Eastern snobbism surfaced defensively.

"I'm used to boring doctors. I don't know if I'm 'mellow' enough to meet your friends."

"Well, I told him about you and he's interested in meeting you. There are other men in the world, my dear."

"I'm sorry, Kate. I know I sound like a whiny child. I just never expected to miss him this way."

"Why don't you go take a nap while I get dinner started. You'll feel better after some rest."

We had just sat down to dinner when Dr. Dan walked in the door. There was a wide grin on his face that spread infectiously around the room. Katrina hugged him and I noticed when she stood next to him how small he was. He wore white pants, sailor pants, a plaid L. L. Bean shirt and a purple vest. His body tilted forward and back as he rocked in wooden clogs, filling his pipe with automatic motions. If it weren't for the pipe I would have never believed he was old enough to have finished medical school. A boyish charm, that was what I detected, but it was unstudied. I caught myself smiling broadly. He reached across the spaghetti to shake my hand. His eyes held me some moments, spilling into mine a sense of childish curiosity, a rare enthusiasm, a desire to play. I could barely recognize it, but I thought I saw happiness in his face. My cheeks reddened in spite of my gloom. I experienced an awkward shyness, an embarrassment, two emotions exiled long ago. After all, a professional woman with an important career, a serious intellectual, cannot afford displays of girlishness. To be honest, however, I had never managed to stifle this quality very well. Seduction was still seductive and I was quite capable of being seduced. He flashed his wide grin at me and there was no mistaking the warm rush into my cheeks.

Dinner continued for hours through several heated conversations from San Diego trivia to the politics of Central America to past acquaintances to medicine. I found myself engrossed in Dan. We argued about everything from antibiotics to vitamins. My tone was unduly aggressive, haughty; it seemed I wanted to offend him. He was as fascinating and intelligent as Katrina had said. I wanted desperately to find something wrong with him, to hear him say something stupid, but he never obliged me. For the moment I had forgotten about Anthony.

The evening was drawing to a close and I lamented about having no place to live. He startled me with a calm "Why don't you move into my house?" This was way too California for me and I guess the look on my face prompted him to qualify the proposition. It was a respectable one. His roommate had recently left, and he wanted to share his rent with someone. The quarters available were two small rooms and a bath. He insisted I could stay there on a trial basis as he was off to Mexico for a week beginning the next day. How ideal, I thought. A nice place to live, a pleasant roommate, I could begin teaching with little worry. It was late, but Dan wanted me to follow him to his house so I could see it before he left. It would be a favor to him, he insisted, if I stayed there and fed the cat. As I drove through the unfamiliar streets, I noticed my sense of dread had lifted. In its place there was an odd excitement, a tingly kind of thrill that annoyed me with its manifestations of a silly smile. It made me feel quite foolish.

I composed myself and inspected the house in a businesslike fashion. Dan stood looking irresistibly cute with his hands in his pockets answering my queries, apologizing for the bathroom, pointing out the fireplace and other amenities. He appeared less certain of himself. There was an atmosphere between us we didn't dare broach. I tried not to look him in the eyes, yet his face was enchanting. A twist of brown hair fell haphazardly over his forehead. A warmth shot through my stomach. I tried to focus on his hands, they were small, constantly in motion. When I asked him about dividing the housework, he pulled his glasses down over his nose and peered at me.

"Perhaps I'll get you a maid." My laughter surprised me, I had forgotten what it felt like to laugh. We stood there laughing together until the time to leave had come and passed. The awkwardness returned. I wished him a pleasant trip, leaving with a glow in my cheeks and a welcomed lightness. Maybe this move was not the end of my life. Maybe it was the beginning of a new one, a life without the struggle, without the endless string of tragedies, without the bleakness of living only because suicide was such a nasty thing to do to others. I could almost forgive myself for the existential philosophy that kept me all too serious and overwrought.

Katrina was asleep when I returned. I crawled into the bed she had set up for me, intensely aware of the excitement between my legs. I wanted Anthony's naked body on top of me. Then I imagined making love to Dan. Banish the thought, I scolded myself.

The next day I moved the contents of my station wagon into his house. It felt different without him and my memories of Anthony filled up the space. I was alone. For days I cried, thinking only of the virtues of solitude. I embraced loneliness and exiled desire. After three days I grew restless and began to clean the house from top to bottom. I reminded myself that Dan was coming back, but I couldn't conceive of him being there. My mattress on the floor symbolized my impoverishment. I would become nunlike and dedicate myself to reading and contemplation. I swore off all men, all sex and absolutely all love. After five days I noticed that I had marked the date of his return on the calendar.

The next day when I was making a foray to the grocery store, a car began honking at me. It was him. What was he doing home early? "See you at home, roomie." His voice was singsong, ebullient, happy. It sounded foreign to me. As I drove to the store my thermometer of panic rose. I wondered if I would throw up. How could I live in that solemn convent with him in the next room? My creation, the tomb, where I mourned Anthony's death, wouldn't accommodate the two of us. Somewhere between the bananas and the avocados I came to my senses. How idiotic this self-serving sorrow! My legs were rubbery, weak, like Jell-O, my stomach embraced a warm rush of pleasure. It was true, I was eager to see him. My desire to see him rose geometrically. Now he was here, there, in his house, our house. I drove to the zoo and sat there thinking that I wasn't a teenager anymore, not even close. I was over thirty, divorced for ten years, not exactly the portrait of Juliet, for God's sake, and yet I believed I was truly jaded where love was concerned. There was no other explanation, it was pure sexual lust. On that manageable note I drove home.

Pots and pans were banging around in the kitchen, jazz blared from the stereo. Dan appeared to be absorbed in cooking. His ear-to-ear smile welcomed me. The house was transformed from my sad cave to a lively home. He had taken my clothes out of the dryer, folded my underwear and hung my slip on a hanger in full view of the kitchen. My pink slip hanging there transported me back to the girlish embarrassment he managed to evoke at our first encounter.

I protested, "You shouldn't have folded my clothes. I'm sorry I left them in the dryer. I didn't expect you until tomorrow."

"Hey, don't worry about it. I decided to come home early and see how you were getting along. I'm the one who should apologize. I see you invested considerable elbow grease in the bathroom. Sorry it was so dirty."

I blushed. "I hope you aren't offended that I cleaned your bathroom. It's the only bathtub, and I'm pretty fussy about bathtubs."

"No, no, don't apologize. I should."

"Don't be silly, it's your house."

"It's our house now." He grinned at me over his glasses.

"What are you making?"

"Bread. I like to bake bread. It's therapeutic. I used to invite my friends over to eat hot bread, but tonight it's late and it won't be ready for a while. Well, how are you? How is everything? Do you like it here?"

"Sure. It's fine. Very comfortable." I stood by the washer feeling useless, wondering how I could get comfortable now that he was back. His wash clicked off, and I automatically put it in the dryer. Men's socks, I couldn't help staring at his socks, his Jockey shorts, size thirty. His sleeves were rolled up as he pounded the dough, his arms were strong, taut, supple, the muscles rippled erotically under the thin shirt. His shoulders were broad, and in the space between them dark hair curled peeking from beneath his shirt. He was tan from a week in the sun. As he chattered about jogging and his daily routine, I thought about his legs. They were short and strong like his arms, perfectly shaped with tight, smooth muscles covered by soft dark hair. I wondered if he always wore jogging shorts at home. Why was he so accessible, enchanting, desirable, sexy? True, he reminded me of Michelangelo's "David," but it was more than his physical appearance. Indeed, I was four inches taller than he, and I had never been attracted to anyone I towered over. I refused to believe in happiness. Surely, whatever it was, it would go away as I got used to him.

He was telling me about his adventures in Mexico, and I was folding his clothes when the doorbell rang. She came into the kitchen before either of us could answer the door. Her dark eyes glowered at me, then turned to Dan. He kissed her on the cheek and introduced us. Relief gushed over me. Of course, I should have known, a handsome, intelligent young doctor wouldn't be without a lover. It was my loneliness, my missing Anthony, that stimulated this shameless attraction to him. How could I have been so egotistical as to imagine he had invited me to live with him for anything other than economic reasons. The relief, I must admit, was mixed with some regret. She ignored me and placed herself in the room directly between Dan and me. I heard her ask him if they could go into the bedroom. It was time to excuse myself. I retreated to my room. The mattress looked emptier than usual. A small photograph of Anthony and me lay beside the bed on the cardboard box I was using for a night table. My briefcase bulged with work to prepare. This was my diversion, yet my ears were tuned for any sounds of passion. Vicarious sex would be better than none at all. I envied her.

A short time later he startled me by knocking on my door and announcing that the bread was ready. I went into the kitchen. She was gone. I didn't ask about her. Instead, we sat on the counters and ate the delicious hot bread with our fingers.

"When will you be home from work tomorrow?" he inquired politely.

"Around five, I guess, my last class ends at four. I need to set up my office and find my way around campus."

"Fine. I'll meet you here and we'll go for a run. Okay? Katrina told me you're a runner."

"Well, I haven't run in weeks, but I suppose I could try. I'm pretty out of shape." I didn't really want to run, but at the moment the urge to be with him dominated. Why did I say that? Why do I want to please him? "I better go to bed now. It's getting late," I said. Leaving the kitchen felt ridiculously difficult. "Goodnight," I added.

"Goodnight." He called after me, "Sweet dreams."

His "sweet dreams" rang in my ears and I hardly slept all night.

For several days I rushed home to find him waiting there. Work was slow at the hospital, he said, but I preferred to think he came home just to see me. We donned our jogging shorts and ran around the city to Balboa Park, the old Mexican part of town, anywhere he hadn't shown me. Afterward, he cooked magnificent Chinese dinners while I sat in a hot bath. One evening I returned to find him on his hands and knees scrubbing the kitchen floor. I wondered if he was this wonderful or if he was doing it for my benefit. The feeling of familiarity grew between us, as did a bittersweet wish for more. Once after a run he patted me on the back and his arm rested on my shoulder just enough for me to feel a burning spot when he took it away. I longed to reach across the dining table and touch his cheek, but we kept ourselves in check, both wondering how to be sure the desires were mutual.

The days were warm, but short. During our long evenings together he made fires after dinner and put soft music on the stereo. We sat quietly and read or talked about unimportant things. In a week we had developed a wonderful routine, the tension, the awkwardness, faded away. The telephone was a nasty intruder. I lay in bed at night reminding myself he was only my housemate, a new friend, a man I hardly knew.

Our first weekend came and we went on a shopping spree to the Payless, piling our cart high with mops, detergents, household gadgets, records and wine. It appeared that we were stocking up for a siege. At the checkout stand he turned and said, "Let's go out for dinner. I know a wonderful little restaurant I'd like to take you to." His hand fell inadvertently on mine.

I didn't move my hand, the softness of his palm was irresistible. "I'd love it." I knew my smile told him how much.

We went home and separately showered and dressed. I wanted to look beautiful and I searched for my most feminine outfit, a white lace blouse and black skirt with tiny rosebuds woven into the soft fabric. The red of my lipstick matched the roses and I added a dash of Tabú to my neck. I emerged from my room tentatively.

He was standing in the living room looking nervous with his hands in his pockets. "You look gorgeous, good enough to eat. Let's hope the food tastes half as delicious as you look."

"You're teasing me, but thanks. Come on, I'm starving."

The restaurant was as romantic as I had imagined, checkered tablecloths, candlelight, fresh flowers. He handed me a daisy to play with until our order came. We were both ravenous and devoured plates piled high with homemade pasta. Before I knew it we were laughing and walking arm in arm toward the car. I was intoxicated with the smell of him and wondered if the red wine had gone to my head. It was late when we arrived home, but neither of us wanted to end the evening. He made a fire and I sat on the floor observing him. I was aware of a tingling sensation that began in my knees and crawled upward toward the inside of my thighs. My heart began to ache for a man's arms around me. I assumed I wanted Anthony. I wanted to touch him, to hold him in my arms, to feel his body naked against mine. Yet I sat thoroughly entranced by Dan, this tireless bundle of energy, this brilliant, handsome, funny kind of doctor who had taken better care of me in one week than anyone else in my entire life. There was no question in my mind about my spiritual devotion to Anthony, but my body kept pulling me elsewhere. Dan got up and returned with a small box.

"You aren't opposed to dope smoking, I hope."

I laughed, "Not at all."

"Great, let's get stoned."

We stared at the fire quite a while, then he turned to me. "You know, since you moved in I haven't seen any of my friends."

"I know, I wondered what happened to your girfriend. I hope I didn't upset anything."

"No, no, that was over long ago anyway. She just needed to talk to me about something."

"Oh." The awkwardness crept up on me. "Well, I don't want to interfere with your social life."

"Not at all. I haven't wanted to see anyone else." His eyes weren't green, I noticed, they were light brown. His lashes were thick and curly. I tried not to stare at him. "I wondered, if you don't mind my asking, what is your relationship with the man in the photograph, Anthony? Are you engaged or something?"

"Oh, no, we're, well, we used to be lovers. But it didn't work out, it's over now. He's committed to living in Boston. I, well, I cared about him a lot, but. . ." I didn't want to discuss the past.

"You mean you're not going back to him?"

"I don't know. I don't know what I'll do or where I'll go. It depends."

"On what?"

Suddenly, I felt light-headed, giggly, like hugging him and blurting out crazy endearments. I let myself turn coy, secretive, seductive and revealing at once. "On whatever may or may not happen here. In California, I mean. I want to explore the West Coast and Mexico; I want to stop spending my life worrying about my career. I want to write novels, travel, have adventures, learn, change. God, I don't know what I want to be when I grow up, and I've already grown up and been some-body." My legs were crossed in a lotus position, and I was staring directly into his eyes as he faced me in the same po-sition. It occurred to me that I had really told him the truth about myself. As soon as I realized it, I wanted to erase it. "God, I guess I've revealed my lack of stability, haven't I? You'd think a college professor would know what she wanted, wouldn't you?" It was hard to impress him when I was stoned. I wasn't sure what impressing him meant anymore. I was acutely aware of his lips.

"I know what I want." He gave me a delicious smile. "I want to kiss you."

"What? Oh. Well, I don't know." He had caught me off guard. My speech was flustered. "I don't think it's a good idea." I was dying to kiss him. "I don't think it's good to mix room-mates and sex. Could lead to all kinds of problems." I was still in control, just barely.

He got up and lit his pipe. "Okay, if that's the way you really feel, but I personally don't see why two consenting unattached adults can't enjoy a kiss by the fire."

"That's not the point. A kiss leads to other things. You know what I mean. Anyway, there's Anthony. I still care about him. How can I kiss you under those circumstances?" My words contradicted the whole thrust of my immediate emotions. I was afraid. If I kissed him it would never stop there.

He was biting his lips as if to hold back laughter. "Do you always analyze everything before you do it? You need to let go of all those tortured little thoughts of yours. You want to kiss me, but you're holding yourself back. It's a disservice to humanity to keep yourself to yourself."

"That sounds very California. I guess I'm not mellow enough yet." I was trying to feel insulted, but he wouldn't have it.

"You're lusciousness itself."

I couldn't resist smiling. I did want to kiss him. He sat back down in front of me and took my hands in his. I felt the warmth of his breath as he slowly leaned over and kissed me, softly, gently, with a measured desire. His lips, full and supple, rested on mine for several moments, then he put his hand on my neck under my hair and pulled my face into his. His tongue met mine and played inside my mouth until this one innocent kiss was as hot as the fire beside us. My arms wanted to fully embrace him, my mouth wished to devour his face, my legs wanted to wrap around his and bring him into me, but, coward that I am, I pulled away.

"I better go to bed now." I retreated to my mattress, shutting the door with a slam. All night I thought of him sleeping down the short corridor, maybe twenty steps away. I tried to think about Anthony, but it didn't work. Again there was no going back. The sky lightened by the time I fell asleep, curled into a ball on my side facing the photograph I refused to put away.

A musky smell of warm maleness filled my senses. My breasts swelled and the nipples grew hard in his hand. A soft moist sensation of lips covered the nape of my neck, then spread to my ears. This was a fabulous dream. A loving hand moved from my breasts to my waist and rested between my thighs. His strong leg went around mine and his kisses crept around to my cheek. An arm slid under me and he turned me toward his body. His cock was swollen between us, I could smell his desire. My arm went naturally around him. My fingers explored the silkiness of his hair, the strength of his shoulders, the shape of his lovely arms, the curvature of his chest, the suppleness of his white bottom. A piercing hot sensation shot up my legs and between them. I wanted him inside me. I wanted to take him in and feel his stomach against mine. He kissed my eyes,

licked my face, my neck, my nipples, until I forgot to realize
that this was not a dream. Our mouths met again, this time
with no reluctance, no hesitation. His kisses were familiar as
if I had been kissing him for years. As he moved me under
him I opened my eyes and saw him, his face ecstatic, his eyes
shimmering, his cheeks red, his brown body poised over mine,
his cock standing up, shining from the silky fluid that dripped
onto my abdomen. He came into me carefully, wrapped his
arms around me and buried his head in my hair. We lay there
together still for some time, his movements began, barely
perceptible. I pressed myself up toward him seeking the in-
comparable pleasure of having him hard inside me for a long
time. With the rhythm of mutual passion, an inability to stay
quiet, our bodies began to move together. The pleasure rose
furiously like the wind before a thunderstorm. He held himself
up on his elbows and looked at me, whispering, "You're incredibly beautiful, you're indescribably lovely, I want to stay
inside you forever." I was speechless, my body burning to keep
him moving in me. The sensation of being completely at his
mercy, of my legs begging to grip him until the pulsing stabs
of pleasure sent me into my own world of total ecstasy. He
sensed my coming, and I heard him crying, whimpering, then
felt the swift spasms of his orgasm, the shooting hot fluid
filling my body. The convulsions subsided, the smell rose between us. He wetly kissed my ears and ran his hands down
my sides, over every inch of my body, and through my hair.
His kisses covered me.

It was a Sunday. We stayed in bed most of the day playing,
making love, talking, eating, reading the paper. On Monday
I put the photograph of Anthony and me away. On Tuesday
he asked me to marry him, and on Wednesday I said yes.

# Malaquite

*UNSIGNED*

We hadn't planned to go to the beach. It was just that Jeff was outraged to hear that I'd been in Texas for three months and had never ventured north to Padre Island, a national seashore.

"All right," I told him, in mock argument, "I'll go next weekend, I promise."

"Why next weekend?" he asked me. "Why not now?"

"Because I'm wearing a skirt and high heels and pantyhose," I explained. We'd been to Corpus Christi to give a presentation to a gathering of various high school groups. We'd been slaving over it together since I'd arrived in Texas. I represented the public affairs office of the university where I worked and he a similar arm of one of the student organizations. He was a senior at the university, but an older senior, twenty-four.

I was forty-two.

We were in his car. We'd agreed to take turns and I had driven up. He was driving back. But he cloverleafed onto Padre Island Drive and headed toward the Gulf Coast.

"We should get something to eat first," he said, pulling into the lot in front of a superette.

I watched him walk away from the car. Actually, I'd been watching him all day and even days before that. He was almost stereotypically gorgeous: more than six feet tall, blond and muscular, though not in any overwrought way. He was wearing a dress shirt, Levi's and cowboy boots. As soon as our presentation had ended, he'd torn off his tie, unbuttoned his shirt and rolled up his sleeves. He was also wearing a thick leather belt with a buckle that read, "Texas." My office could have

85

used him on campus recruiting posters.

He came back with a brown paper bag and a six-pack of beer. "You know what?" he said, pushing the groceries toward me on the seat, "I think I have a couple blankets in the trunk. I'll go see." He pulled the keys from the ignition and went around to the back of the car. He returned with a heap of army green. He tossed the heap into the back seat. "This'll be nice," he said.

"Wait a sec," I told him, getting out of the car and heading toward the superette. "I need cigarettes." I'd managed to quit more than a month ago, but I did, right then, need cigarettes. I bought three packs.

"I thought you quit," he said, when I eased myself back into the car. I had told him that on the way up.

"This is just in case," I answered.

He turned the radio on, opened a can of beer and handed it to me. I took a sip and he retrieved it, stashing it between his legs. "We'll share it," he told me, "okay?" He looked at me over his sunglasses, which were low on his nose.

"Okay."

He pushed the glasses back into place and we drove on, nearing the bridge that spanned the Intracoastal Waterway. There was shallow water on both sides, white dots on the water.

"Look over there," he said, gesturing. "Pelicans." Several of the white dots rose up flapping, as if he'd cued them. I laughed. "Trained them myself," he laughed with me. "It wasn't easy."

I looked down at the beer. He saw me looking. "Go ahead," he said, lifting his elbows and making his legs part a little wider. I reached for the beer can, careful not to touch him. I wasn't immune to him, physically. I only thought that he might be immune to me. After all, no amount of yoga and riding and swimming and racquetball could negate my age.

The road narrowed. There were sand dunes on either side. We passed a sign giving the distance to Malaquite Beach. "That's where I'm taking you," he said.

I had, for the past month, been dating another man. He was a suitable man, divorced, successful, forty-four. He never "took" me anywhere, but asked, always, where I would like to go. I chose restaurants, usually.

"What did you get to eat?" I started rummaging through the brown bag. Apples. Bananas. A can of nuts. Two Hershey bars.

"Don't eat that now," Jeff said. "Save it till we get there." Then he turned the radio up and we drove the rest of the way just listening to it. Rock: Rod Stewart. Fleetwood Mac. Heart.

He pulled into the parking lot of Malaquite. There were no other cars. "Why isn't anyone out here?" I asked him.

"It's a weekday," he explained. "And anyway, it'll be getting cold." He leaned over the seat to get the blankets. I started out of the car. "Uh-uh," he said. "You have to take your shoes off, remember? And your pantyhose."

I kicked my shoes off, then stood outside the car to wiggle out of my hose. He didn't even try to watch, though I watched him remove his boots, his socks, then roll his jeans so that his calves were exposed.

"Get the groceries," he told me, taking the blankets and the remaining cans of beer.

The sun was setting, but not on the Gulf side where we might have seen it. There was a wide band of yellow back beyond the dunes. We turned away from it and walked, side by side, toward the sea.

I could hear the waves from the moment we'd quit the car. Nonetheless, I caught my breath when I saw them. Rows and rows and rows. And close to each other, too, so that the sound was constant rather than rhythmic.

"I feel that way too," he said, having heard me gasp. "Every time I come here."

We stepped off the pavement and onto the sand. Bits of shell and nettle jabbed at the soles of my feet. I took maybe four steps and started ouching out loud.

"A tenderfoot," he teased me. "I should have known."

I had a fleeting wish that he would sweep me into his arms and carry me to the water's edge. And then we would be Deborah Kerr and Burt Lancaster, *From Here to Eternity*. Instead he offered, "Tell you what. I'll walk in front of you and you can walk in my footsteps, okay?"

His footsteps were huge and much too far apart for me to step with ease from each to each. "Step smaller," I told him, and he laughed at me but did so. And his method worked. The sand where he had stepped was smoother, all mashed down.

"Why doesn't it hurt *your* feet?" I asked him, shouting to be heard above the waves.

"Because I've been doing this forever," he called back to me.

I almost believed that he meant it literally. That we were enacting some primordial scene. I turned and looked at the Malaquite pier to remind myself that this was now.

"Here's a good place," he said, spreading one of the blankets. He knelt on it and removed his shirt. I watched the goose-bumps form on his shoulders and his back. I wanted to touch his back, the way I'd wanted to touch his thigh when I'd reached for the beer. I would have to be careful not to.

"What's the matter?" he asked me, patting the blanket so that I would sit.

"Nothing." I sat and put the grocery bag off to the side.

He took his sunglasses off and leaned back, clasping his hands behind his head. He closed his eyes.

That meant I could look at the whole of him without his knowing it, and I did, thinking all the while of what I'd like to do. Run my hands through the hair on his chest. Draw my fingertips across his shoulders. Unhitch that Texas belt buckle. Unzip his jeans.

Why didn't I?

Because I was afraid. That he'd laugh at the notion of someone my age. That he'd laugh again later, telling his friends. Or worst of all, that he'd tell me, with great seriousness, how I'd misunderstood and how he hadn't meant to lead me on. That this was simply a neighborly introduction to the beach.

But I really wanted to take his hand and say, Jeff? Did it occur to you that I'm wearing absolutely nothing underneath this skirt?

"That picture in your office," he said, opening his eyes. "Who is that?" He'd been to my office nearly twice a week since my tenure here began.

"My son."

"How old is he?" he asked.

"You don't want to know," I said, laughing and moving a couple more inches away.

"How old? Tell me."

"Twenty-one."

"I'm twenty-four," he said.

"I know."

He sat up. "Does that bother you?" he asked me. "Because if it doesn't. . ." He dropped back onto the blanket, the rest of the sentence unsaid. He'd closed his eyes again.

I knelt beside him, my skirt slightly raised, my bare knees on the wool of the blanket. "You're leaving this up to me?"

He smiled, but didn't open his eyes, didn't move, didn't anything.

I looked around to make sure that we were still alone out there. We were.

"All right," I said. "I'd like to look at you. Without these." I pinched at the seam of his Levi's.

He laughed and reached for his buckle.

"And let me do it," I said.

He lifted his hips, though, to help slide the jeans over them. I pulled his pants completely off. He wasn't wearing any underwear.

He had a wonderful erection. I wanted to touch it, wanted to suck on it, wanted to push my skirt all the way up and lower myself over it.

Instead, I chickened out altogether. I swiveled and groped toward the edge of the blanket for another beer. "Jeff." I tried to sound as if I were kidding him. "Is this one of your fantasies? To have some woman maul all over you while you just lie there with your eyes shut?" I had my rear end toward him while I spoke and was busily trying to pop the top of the can. I got it part of the way off.

"That's pretty close," he said. He'd gotten up. He was pushing at my skirt from behind and when my ass was bare, he let his body cover mine. I felt his penis between my legs and the hair around his penis against my backside. "But not the 'some woman' part," he said. He might have meant several women all at once. On the other hand, he might have meant just me. He leaned forward and kissed the back of my neck just above my collar. His kiss was soft and damp and made me shiver. I pressed myself against him and felt his penis, not inside me but against me. It was wet all over, wet from me.

I set the beer can down and it tipped. The beer started dribbling onto the sand.

"Stay on the blanket," he told me, moving back toward the center. He leaned back again and watched as I moved toward him on my knees. He put his hand between my legs, pushing the hem of my skirt as high as he could. He played with me and didn't stop when I squirmed to lie beside him. I moved my hand over his testicles and his sticky penis. We kissed for the longest time, touching each other that way.

It was totally dark now, and it had, as he'd said it would, grown cold. He pulled the second blanket over us. "I want to take my clothes off," I said. He told me I would freeze to death, but helped me. Then we snuggled underneath the scratchy wool.

He teased me with his penis, letting it poke between my legs or enter me just a bit before he'd pull away.

"Damn you," I said, "would you *please*—"

"Would I please what?"

But then he entered me a little more. "Please do this?" he asked me. A little more. "This?"

Only our heads stuck out from underneath that blanket, and occasionally, by mistake, his feet. Then he'd swear at the blanket, and whirl it back around and into place. I had sand in my hair and sand stuck to my cheek.

Part of the time we were quiet and sweet with each other and part of the time we were not. Part of the time, we'd fool around, fucking a little and then stopping, kissing, licking, tickling, touching.

"What do you call this technique of yours?" I asked him.

"Little of this, little of that," he said.

He made me come with his fingers and with just the tip of his penis against my clitoris. Then he made me come with his penis deep inside.

He moved behind me, spoon style. He entered me again. He wet his fingers with the juices that were running down my thigh and rubbed at my breasts and my nipples. "What a sticky little pussy you have," he whispered in my ear. Just the flow of his breath might have made me come again. I pushed back at him, wanting him as deep as he could go. Wanting to feel his balls brushing against me, too. He came inside me that way, from behind. We were contentedly still until his penis slithered out on its own. We sat up then, and munched our fruit and nuts and chocolate and guzzled our beer. We talked about all the stars and how neither of us had noticed them during.

But it was a weekday. We had to start back. It must be, I deduced, long past midnight. We gathered up our things and trudged toward the car. I felt wonderful. Every now and then I could smell his come. Could he?

I didn't want to ask. But then I didn't have to. Just before he opened the car door, he stood close to me and whiffed and smiled and said, "Hmmm."

Inside the car, we didn't speak, didn't turn the radio on. We did hold hands when he wasn't shifting gears. But before we got off the island, he pulled into another parking lot. A Holiday Inn. "What are you doing?" I asked him.

"Shhh," he said. "It's just another fantasy. But you have to keep your mouth shut."

We walked up a path and alongside a lighted, glassed-in building. There was a security guard inside. He was reading something. We went past the building he was in and up a little flight of concrete stairs. There was an outdoor Jacuzzi at the top, bubbling away. I looked up at the hotel and nearly all the rooms were dark.

I was a little dizzy from all the beer, though he'd drunk most of it. It was hard to keep from laughing.

We undressed and slipped into the heated water.

"I stayed here once with my parents," he whispered. "Compared to this, it wasn't any fun."

He reached up over the side and fished something out of his shirt pocket. It was a joint. We shared it, and afterward just let our bodies silk against each other in the little pool.

All those stars again. "The same ones," he said.

Then he made the "shhh" sign at me with his finger and got out of the water, running naked along the path. I kept my eye on the lighted building where the guard was. I had a flash vision of being arrested for trespassing, possession of marijuana and dallying with a college-aged youth. It only made me laugh. I had to duck myself under the water, in fact, because I was laughing out loud.

Jeff came back with the blankets.

He made one into a cushion and set it on the Jacuzzi's edge. Then he got down into the water and lifted me up to sit on the cushion he'd made. "Put the other one around you," he instructed, and I took the second blanket and did so. He stood in the water in front of me and put my feet on his shoulders. He put his head between my legs and my feet slid down his back. He licked me and kissed me and sucked me and blew his breath against me. Narrow, cool streams and big, hot puffs.

"My God, Jeff," I said. He pulled away and let his arms rest atop my thighs.

"I told you," he said, "you have to keep your mouth shut."

I heard the glass doors slide open. I heard the security guard's footsteps coming closer. Jeff went back to licking me, but not all over as he had been doing. Only my clitoris now. The footsteps stopped. Went past. Returned. Finally, I heard the glass doors slide shut again. "You bastard," I whispered.

Jeff made his tongue as flat as he could. I could hear how wet I was. "I knew I could make you come again," he said. I shook myself out of the blanket and slid back down into the water. We hugged each other and laughed as quietly as we could. "Of course, a little terror never hurts," he said, looking over at the guard's place.

We got back nearly at dawn. There was a note stuck to my screen. From my sensible man. "Hoped to catch you for dinner," it read. "Perhaps tomorrow? Hope all went well in Corpus."

"Well," Jeff said, kissing my fingertips, "didn't it?"

But I didn't want the night to end. And anyway, I had to be in my office at eight, so what point was there in going to sleep?

"That does make some sense," Jeff told me.

Inside, he examined the contents of my fridge. "Okay, you just sit back and take it easy," he announced.

He made taquitos: flour tortillas with scrambled egg and melted cheese and red hot piquante sauce inside. And coffee, thick and black. I leaned back in a chair while I ate and dribbled red sauce all over the front of my already grungy blouse.

He was sitting on the hassock.

"What a slob you are," he laughed, setting his empty plate aside and taking mine to put atop it. He stood up, tucked his thumbs behind his belt. "You like to eat, don't you? I'll bet you're still hungry." There was a lot of tease in his eyes and his voice. I put my hands on his ass and tugged him toward me.

He kicked the hassock aside and unhitched his belt, undid his zipper, slid his jeans down over his hips. I caught his erection in my mouth. It seemed wonderfully raunchy except for the way he stroked my hair.

Eventually, we found our way into my bedroom, though not to sleep. I did make my eight-o'clock office appointment and he his eight-o'clock class.

But that isn't the end of the story.

Jeff was showering when I told him I'd been asked to write a true piece of erotica. He pulled the shower curtain to the side and dripped all over the edge of the tub. "That ought to be easy," he said. "Just write about you and me. That first night. What's it been now?" counting in his head. "How about that. It's been four months."

He reached out with his wet arm and pulled at the sash of my robe. "Hey, come on," he said. Then he stepped back under the water jet. The curtain was still open wide.

The water streamed all over his face, bounced off his shoulders and his head. It splashed all over the bathroom, too. "Are you going to stand out there and take your shower?" he asked me. "Or are you going to come in here? With me."

# II

# QUALITIES OF
# EROTIC MOMENTS

Beyond the emotional relationship, there are numerous other factors that account for making a sexual experience memorable. Some of these qualities are as simple as anticipation or playfulness, the nature of the setting or the basic sensations of the physical experience. Other qualities are more complex. Sometimes an experience is erotic because of the power of dynamics in the relationship; other times it is erotic because the unexpected has occurred, something so totally unplanned that the other person, the sex and the relationships involved are transformed by the experience.

## Anticipation

Routine can relegate sex to the ranks of the mundane. Not giving sex a high priority often means that it assumes the position of least importance in a relationship, occurring late at night after the chores are completed, the children are asleep and very little time and energy are left over. Keeping a sexual relationship vital requires time and attention. Sometimes this can be done by setting aside special evenings or weekends to be together and planning for sex in a way that allows the anticipation to build. By making sex special it becomes something to look forward to, setting in motion a mental foreplay that can enhance and intensify the actual experience.

Reunions after periods of time spent apart are automatically imbued with this special sense of anticipation. In the story "Sailing Away," the author is accustomed to frequent and long separations. Being married to a man who spends much of his time at sea means that she often looks forward to the few hours they can steal away together. While not a life-style most couples would choose, these circumstances do make the time together sexually charged. According to the author, "It's always been like this. He'll be gone for two months at a clip and there will be so little time together that every moment is special. Because we're united so infrequently, this kind of sex adds to the relationship and makes it incredibly intense. I still feel that way and we've been married for ten years."

Dorothy Schuler had infrequent encounters with her lover for different reasons. During the five-month period upon which "Siblings" is based, Dorothy was married and could only slip away for infrequent clandestine meetings. But even after her marriage ended, she and her lover continued to see each other only occasionally. This, she felt, not only suited his personality but made their time together something to look forward to. In her words, "We saw each other inconsistently—sometimes only once every two weeks, sometimes more often. When we did, it was a step outside of time, an escape from reality. A lot was happening in both our lives, and we didn't discuss those things: I didn't even tell him when I left my husband. The occasionality of it made being together a treat, like a strawberry dipped in chocolate, but you don't want to eat too many. Because I didn't see him too often, we had time to anticipate each other and our time together."

Sometimes the anticipation can be as good as or better than the actual sexual experience. Mary Beth Crain, the author of "Picasso," will never know, because anticipation was the only aspect she ever experienced in a relationship with a man much older than herself. Yet the verbal innuendos and sexual tension permeated the relationship over a period of years. "He was a master of verbal foreplay," she told me. "I had certain needs, and he filled them. At the time, I felt that I wasn't getting enough attention from my husband and I needed to feel attractive again as a woman. The man in the story was very sophisticated and sexually oriented. He exuded an enjoyment of sex that took it out of the realm of the ordinary and into the dimension of art. A lot of the erotic part of our relationship was my expectation of how uninhibited he would be in bed. He liked to talk about the art of lovemaking to titillate me and, in a certain way, he was bringing out my dark side—feelings I was afraid of but which were exciting in a good, fun, creative way. His being older also added to the fantasy of his being the sexual expert."

A different aspect of anticipation is illustrated by Signe Hammer. In fact, in her story, "1968," the sense of expectation and anticipation forms the entire erotic component as she leaves the consummation of the sexual experience with this absolute stranger totally to our imagination. "I don't find explicit sexuality erotic," says Signe. "So this story is very oblique, like the chess game in *The Thomas Crown Affair*, which is one of the most erotic things I've ever seen on film. Explicit sex gets to be repetitious. The breast is kissed, the camera moves down to the genitals. Actually, most of the time, explicit sex is just funny. When the approach is oblique, the possibilities are infinite. The erotic thing about sexuality, I think, is the expectation."

Signe believes, however, that men and women differ in their response to anticipation. "Men want to get right to the point," she says. "A man's response is rapid; that's inherent in the nature of male sexuality. Sometimes it's hard for men to realize that women are different, that we need more than just the sight and awareness of their bodies to become aroused." In reference to her story, she says, "I think the fact that the pleasure is in the anticipation would make many men impatient with this piece. I am dwelling on the intermediate details. The only male who did this was Henry James, and he was known for never getting on with it."

### Playfulness and Humor

Many people find the ability to play in bed and to treat sex with humor essential ingredients to enjoyable sex. To these people, sex is best not when it is silent and serious but when it is more like a form of grown-up play. When it can be adventurous, when joking and laughter are part of the process, it becomes more exciting and more satisfying. This was the attitude shared by the four authors whose stories are included in this section.

The therapist who authored "The Fifty-Minute Hour: Between the Minutes..." sees sex as "good, clean fun. I chose these stories because there was risk-taking plus humor." She told me, "It was all so spontaneous and unplanned that it captured the imagination. There was no spoken agreement to do something crazy, but my partner and I were both up for something spontaneous at the same time. There was also the risk of getting caught and the sense of wanting to flaunt it. Here we were grown-ups and we could do whatever we wanted. It was like putting something over on someone. And not only was it erotic, but we laughed a lot."

The author who wrote "How I Spent My Summer Vacation" feels that sex is best when it is most spontaneous and uncontrolled. "That summer was a real adventure because I could be out of control and open with everyone," she says. "This is not the norm for me. I'm generally a very controlling person. But when I relinquish the control, incredible things happen. That summer, it was like I had a sign on my back that said 'Fuck me.' I was exuding some kind of energy that told people I was available and I think that had something to do with the fact that I felt ready for anything. I could be totally outrageous, and it was fun."

The sense of playfulness and adventure also comes through in "Truckin'" by Brooke Newman. Without ever making contact with her fantasized partner, she managed to create a wonderfully erotic game. What makes this story even more interesting is that Brooke was eight months pregnant when the incident took place. According to Brooke, "Nothing seems very erotic when you're pregnant except possibly sitting in an automobile where the other person doesn't know you're pregnant. Otherwise, no one would ever look twice. When this story occurred, I was on my way to my lawyer's office to make out my will. There is something very exciting about making out your will, if you take it seriously. It is the one time you can say anything you please to anyone, so I was up for something that day. Driving to my attorney's office and considering the possibility that I might not be immortal made it all the more exciting. There was a baby kicking inside my belly and a truck driver 'at my door.' There was the fantasy of the person behind the wheel, and the playing back and forth together. All I could see were his gigantic arms, tattoos and face; a shiny black truck, the huge wheels; it was an eighteen-wheeler (and the wheels were as tall as my Jeep). The bridge we crossed was sensual as it undulated over the water, and it was exciting to move along at high speeds above the San Francisco Bay—not bad for an eight-months-pregnant woman."

Grace Zabriskie, who authored "Screaming Julians," takes a similar kind of game and moves it from the physical to the verbal level. For Grace, one aspect of eroticism involves continuing a conversation, "a teasing and/or somewhat witty one," throughout sexual play. She says, "Although I sometimes really want to be quiet and make love, I also like creating this tension through continuing the dialogue. But it has to be a mutual conspiracy. It takes two people playing the game at once to make it work." Grace feels that this kind of humor and repartee are important factors to some women's sexual arousal. "Women should know that verbal communication and humor during sex can be wonderful. We shouldn't feel weird if we like it. Also, men should know this about us. The second Screaming Julian knew this about me and went one better. He knew how to play verbally, and even how to chide me about my verbalness in a way that prolonged and enhanced our lovemaking."

### The Physical

For some people, the physical sensitivities and bodily sensations form the primary focus of the sexual encounter. In some ways the images created by poetry are best suited for describing this physical aspect of lovemaking. In "The Work to Know What Life Is," Deena Metzger penetrates into the depth of the physical experience without shyness or a sense of physical denial. For Deena, lovemaking is "being within nature, an act so natural and lacking in self-consciousness that it goes beyond the act itself." And this is how she portrays it in her poem.

"The Drainage Ditch" also sustains itself on the intensity of the physical experience by accentuating all of the senses to their fullest. For the author, this incident was a fantasy come true. "I had fantasies of making love outdoors, but I had never done it because of burrs or stickers or mosquitoes," she said. "But in this unlikely place, with mud everywhere except on our hands, which had been covered by gloves, it was wonderful. The experience of doing physical labor and the smell of springtime made the experience extraordinary. Even the sound of the mud sucking at our boots was sensuous. And the fact that it was a fantasy lived out made it much richer."

## The Context

The context, both the mental frame of mind and the environmental setting, can elicit the truly erotic. Making love outdoors or changing the usual room or bed can add novelty and increase passion. For the author of "Tropical Places," the setting was the key to her erotic adventures, not only because the places themselves were sensual but because being in physical environments which were free from the stresses and constraints of her daily work world enabled her to open up parts of herself which she truly enjoyed and through which she could fully engage in the erotic experience. According to the author, "These experiences were among my shortest affairs, but they are vivid in my memory because of the setting. The environment provided a certain music and fragrance, and there were palm trees and sun. This kind of mood and setting bring out a special part of myself that I really like and that men find attractive. I didn't have to worry about whether my mascara was in place, there were no stockings, girdle, makeup, no answering service. I'm more sensual and comfortable when half clothed than in a gabardine suit. I felt no pressure because I knew the relationship was temporary. I didn't have to worry about being too forward and waiting for the third date, because there would be no third date. I couldn't fantasize and put unrealistic expectations on the man. There were no worries about children, other girlfriends, his emotional stability, and as a result I could be much more relaxed and fully in the moment."

It is also possible to transform a sexual experience without moving an inch. Through fantasy, we can enter a totally new and exciting terrain—the terrain of the imagination—and the lovemaking can take on characteristics far beyond the physical reality. Deena Metzger based her story "The Bull Dancer" on such a sexual experience in which she is clearly transported to another reality. According to Deena, "There was a chemistry that moved the experience onto a mythic level. I was making love but felt simultaneously that I was the moon queen visited by the bull god. This element of fantasy moved physiology another dimension into myth. It was a step up from theater, beyond the senses. It was cosmic or spiritual sex, an altered state of consciousness."

### Power

Capitalizing on the various aspects of power in a relationship can intensify a couple's lovemaking. Dominance and submission are forms of sexuality that pervade the literature and many people's sexual fantasies. In the extreme, we find sadism and masochism such as that explored in *Story of O* by Pauline Réage, but in less intense forms we see other kinds of power dynamics at play. Using power to make the interaction more sexually exciting is something some couples enjoy toying with. And while preferences for the dominant and submissive role vary, both positions can be equally powerful. The traditional power role is described by Carol Conn in "A Few Words on Turning Thirty in Marin County, California," while the role of the one who really allows the dominant one to dominate is explored in "And After I Submit."

Totally controlling her two male slaves, Carol Conn enjoys the power of having every whim indulged. She has created a real-life fantasy that has a decadent eroticism all its own. According to Carol, "I created the feeling of being totally overwhelmed and catered to, of total sensual selfishness. It was like having a genie in a lamp who could make any wish come true, like having the power of royalty."

In "And After I Submit," the man is ostensibly the more powerful one in the relationship. But according to the author, his strong need for her gave her tremendous power. "The intensity of the feelings between us was great, but power was always an issue," she said. "His drive was to always be in total control of the situation. I find dominant masculine power to be very exciting, and the fact that he had that kind of power turned me on. But while this power was attractive, it was also dangerous because he wanted to break my will. He used dominant forceful power, but I used sexual energy. He was totally dependent on getting that from me, and that's where I had *my* power. The story really shows the transmutability of power, the way that each person can use it to its full erotic potential."

### Transformation

Sometimes a sexual experience is so unique it can transform a person's life. When very close and long-term platonic friendships become sexual, even just one time, the effect can be profound. The willingness to relinquish expectations, to step beyond boundaries that assume friendships are one way and sexual relationships another and to trust that the friendship will survive regardless of the outcome of the sexual experience has, for some people, led to peak experiences. Two authors chose to write about sexual experiences that occurred with close and longtime friends, experiences they felt had had a deep and transformative impact on their lives.

For Syn Ferguson, the eroticism conveyed in "Prisoners" is merely one part of a bond of friendship she shared with two men while they were all in the military. The transformation for Syn occurred when she entered into the sex not out of her own needs but as a favor to the two men. She never imagined that the result would be such a total and deep-felt experience. According to Syn, "At no great sacrifice to myself, I was trying to do Bela and Paul a favor. I didn't expect anything. I wasn't thinking about myself; I'm usually evaluating my performance during sex, rating my partner, etc. Bela was also intently focused on Paul. Because we were both less self-conscious, the result was a cosmic explosion that exceeded ordinary consciousness. If that's not spiritual, I don't know what is."

For Jacquie Robb, "The Growing Season" transformed her life because she was able to remain friends with Nancy even after their sexual relationship ended. Their friendship helped her to leave a rural environment and reach out to new experiences. Previously, if a sexual relationship hadn't worked out, Jacquie would never have seen the person again. "This relationship," she said, "was radically different. I could have felt rejected, and part of me wanted to feel this way, but another part of me realized that it didn't matter whether or not we were sexual, and that was new for me. I felt good about how I dealt with the situation, and now we have a real solid friendship. The whole experience helped me realize that it's possible to have a long-term friendship with someone I had been sexual with. Also, because of our solid love, I had the confidence to leave Maine, where I had been living, and do what I wanted to do."

These qualities—anticipation, playfulness, humor, the setting, the physical and the mental stimulation—can account for creating truly erotic moments, as the authors in this section clearly illustrate.

# ANTICIPATION

## Sailing Away

### UNSIGNED

I knew Von was coming into port soon with his ship, the *Medina*, but I didn't know the exact day. He is thirty-one and works as a mate for an East Coast oil company. My husband, my lover, my friend. Though I should be accustomed to it by now, I am invariably a little taken by surprise when he calls. Of course that decidedly adds to our excitement—our anticipation of being together again at last.

We met in the late afternoon at the ship terminal, a windswept pier from which we had a fine view of the moon rising in the blue celestial sphere over the bay. He wore loosely fitted ivory muslin sailing pants and a richly woven ivory cotton sweater. As we embraced, I recognized the rustling of his pants against my thighs. He kissed my lips, a long lingering kiss. In that instant, weakness took me in the knees, my heart faint with lust to lie beside him.

"How was your drive?" he asked, his voice smoky, with the wind blowing it softly to my ears.

"Nice. As always, I've had butterflies since you called," I answered, smiling into his eyes.

Pleased with this, he smiled, his head gracefully inclined toward me, filling my eyes with his powerful beauty. Tall lithe beauty, head to foot. Massive shoulders with soft curls—like petals of wild roses, all brassy brown. Smooth, peachy complexion, somewhat ruddy with sun. Gently slanting, dark, yet clear brown eyes, evenly set, with a straight nose. A man with the classic image of a Greek god.

"I haven't had much sleep, so you can drive," he said as we got into the car.

"How long do we have together?" I searched his eyes.

"About thirty hours is all," his mind ranging.

"Thirty hours of treasure," I said, making the best of it. "Have you had supper yet?" I asked as we drove along the causeway.

"No," he said. "I want to take you out."

I asked, "What would you like then?"

Von looked at me, his jawline solemn, and said, "You." Then he clasped my wrist. "It's so good to see you."

Looking from the road to his eyes, and then down his body, I agreed. "I know. I missed you too." Impulsively, I reached over and ran my hand easily down his crotch. He gasped lightly, delighted by the gesture. My hand lingered and felt him respond beneath it. Our eyes met. He told me not to stop; I pressed down. As I ran my hand smoothly back and forth over the fabric, I felt the strength and power of the rod beneath. I sensed a rush of electric current between my legs, a strong pulse.

Straining to keep my eyes on the road, I wriggled in my seat and opened the sun roof. The clean breeze refreshed my skin.

Again I let my eyes look his way. He clasped my hand, put it to his lips and kissed it. He put it down to rest on his leg and readily unfastened his pants, revealing his bold penis.

Instinctively, I put my hand on it, around it, and finally

beneath it. I lifted it a little; I let my eyes fall to it. His penis appeared polished where the sunlight fell upon him. I felt the smoothness, the density of the shaft.

Ordinarily he wears silky bikini underwear. I observed, "You aren't wearing underwear today, babe."

Smiling, he said, "I'll bet you aren't either."

Beneath my flannel skirt and blouse was my bare skin. I felt exquisitely sexy, giving him an innocent smile.

I caressed his penis as we rode along and talked lightly, with mingled sighs of growing passion.

"How was New York?" I asked as we walked in the door.

"Oh, it was great. I went to Greenwich Village, ate at a quaint little Italian place and went to see *Gandhi;* you should definitely see it." Then, "I brought you some things," taking them out of the bag one by one, "a *Village Voice,* the February issue of Andy·Warhol's *Interview,* a pretty card and chopsticks for your hair."

I thanked him with eager affection.

Setting all else aside, we made our way to our bedroom. "It is good to be home, love," he said as he began to remove his clothes. "Our bed looks inviting."

We recently bought a wonderful waveless waterbed with an oak headboard which has an oval mirror with an ornate etching on it. A thick seascape comforter covers the water mattress and frame.

I undressed while Von went to put on some music. I looked up; he stood naked beyond the door, in plain sight. I seized the moment to admire his excellent body. Supple, lean and young. Handsome, delicate feet and ankles, with rich thighs— like a hurdler's. A taut, flat stomach molding upward to his dense rib cage and upper arms. Very smooth skin, very enticing.

As we reached for each other, Von grasped my wrist; touched my arms, my shoulders. With unutterable joy we got onto the bed facing one another, hand in hand, eye to eye. He rolled onto his back as I turned onto him, kissing him, touching him, moving downward. He sighed with pleasure as I consumed him. His sighing provoked my own desire for him. I looked up into the mirror at the reflection of my mouth and his penis. "Ooh, I love that," he whispered. He rolled his head to one side softly, touched in a bit of laughter. There is nothing that my lover does not notice.

He tipped his fingers upon my shoulders, saying, "Come here." His loving words reached my loving ears in soft whispers.

I moved toward him, knowing he was a little weary. He held me, kissed me. Gently rolling us over, he said, "And now, for your pleasure."

"You are my pleasure, babe."

He traced my face under his spread hands, telling me he loved me. We kissed long, passionately, gyrating with desire for each other. His tender mouth enveloped my nipples, sucking gently while his tongue teased the very tips. My breasts swelled in excitement.

He moved slowly down my body, kissing me softly with his lips and tongue. His golden fingers sliding over me, touching me, caressing, gently squeezing.

He took my foot in his hands and put my toes to his lips. Kissing them, sucking them, moving his tongue erotically between them.

He then moved upward, between my legs, turning his head to kiss the inside of my knees. He spread my legs apart and ran his fingers smoothly up my thighs. Lightly touching me, spreading my vagina, he put his loving lips and tongue to me.

His breath warm, light chills spread over my body as he caressed me with his mouth. In a peak of passion, he brought me to rhythmic orgasm.

With insatiable desire, I wrapped my legs around his shoulders. His mouth eagerly responded to my embrace, engulfing me completely. Beneath his lips and tongue I quivered into a crescendo of luscious orgasms.

He held me close, each of us loving that ultimate feeling of closeness, that tranquillity.

We showered together, bathing one another completely with sweet soap. As we held each other closely, he said, "Our bodies are perfect together."

We chose to eat oysters on the half shell—that renowned aphrodisiac—at the Black Diamond Raw Bar. We each had oysters and beer, though not too much, for we would never want to be too full for love. It was very intimate. Von kissed me and said, "To look at us, one would never think we've been married for ten years." He truly knows just the perfect thing to say.

On the way home Von asked, "Should I stop and get us some wine?"

"No, I have champagne chilled for you, as always."

Von filled wineglasses while I changed into the gown he had given me for Christmas. Transparently lavender, soft, silky, sensuous. He delights in my wearing it.

Making some time to talk is always especially important to us, because of our life-style, his work. We spend many hours talking and loving, nurturing our relationship.

After telling each other the trials of our separation, we talked of a future full of promise. We sat close, in bed, our legs entwined.

We love using the romantic effect of candles. Filling the air with Eden scents: sandalwood, vanilla, jasmine.

The candlelight cast a radiance over him, his salty voice caressed me, intoxicating me.

"How 'bout a massage?" I asked, longing to caress him, to breathe the heavenly fragrance that came from him.

"For me or you?" he responded.

"For you, babe, just for you." I smiled in reply.

A smile came then to his lips; he looked at me and said, "I'd love it."

He turned poetically onto his stomach, in front of the mirror.

I spread my legs and straddled his loins, my gown falling to our sides. I then poured oil liberally into my palms, warming it between them.

Anointing his back and shoulders completely, I sensed the intimacy beneath my palms and fingers. I worked my palms into his lean steadfast muscles, feeling the tension dissolve, his silken skin sleek with rich oil. With each stroke upon his extensive brown shoulders I felt a surge of excitement.

He opened his heavy eyes and looked up into the mirror at me. I took my gown off, drawing it up over my head, my hair falling in wild disarray. He gasped in sensational seductive exclamation.

Smiling, I lay down on his back, my nipples pressing to his satin skin. He let out a passionate groan. I slid my hands beneath him to his stomach. Skating my fingers over him, his hair like lace.

I rolled off him, gently turning him to me, my hand still at his navel. I moved my hand freely up his broad torso, and then down the inside of his inclining thigh. I leaned to him, brushing my lips over his stomach to his welling penis.

I stretched my arms out to clasp his shoulders. His right hand touched my throat, his left hand pulled me near. Our parted lips met, playing so tenderly and erotically.

I moved onto him.

So effortlessly—in one motion I lifted his penis into me. We moved with each other, for each other. Leaning onto his heaving chest, I felt his breath upon my neck. We turned easily onto our sides. Aroused to fresh zeal, giving to each other in rhythm and melody, surrendering a rich perfume. As I quivered with intense orgasms, he filled me with his hot succulent nectar.

Mingled in love, charmed to stillness, in each other's arms we lay.

He turned onto me, kissing me with his rose lips, and said, "Oh, how I love you," his fingers gently brushing across my cheek.

Then, still at last, with the honey-salt air, we slept in peace. Our bodies relaxed, rest was sweet for us.

After the pleasure of love and sleep, I awakened to the treasure in my arms. My man, a luxury.

I lay there for an hour, holding him, indulging myself in his beauty. Afraid to fail my lover, I tried to decide just how to wake him, wanting to give him special pleasure.

Too late, I saw him just waking from sleep. Troubled by a dream, he whispered, "Just hold me, love."

After a while he squeezed me, saying, "Let's go watch the sunrise together."

"That sounds perfect," I replied, knowing our time together was nearing an end.

Von started our bath, and soon we slipped into the cool delicious water. I leaned to him, my back against his chest, both reveling in little chatter.

So worn in love and thought, we bathed our fair bodies, soothing our brows.

We dressed warmly for the brisk morning air on the bay. I

filled big mugs full of hot chocolate laced with cinnamon, to take along.

We parked on the seawall and walked down to the beach, with the breath of wind upon us. The sunrise twilight danced on our silhouettes, the whole heaven seemed a part of us.

With the breakers' sigh on the beach, dawn met us at the shore—holding one another, gazing toward the horizon. Von's name was on my lips when, with the first daylight, he kissed me. The light overwhelmed the sky, winds buffeted the gales of our voices.

We drove slowly from the waterfront to the ship channel, time running out.

We stood on the dock by the ship. The wind stirred up some spirit in my heart. Von cast me a glance. It was time. The wind pierced my heart. I stood in panic. He took me in his arms.

"Don't cry," he said. "Just love me."

Joy and anguish took my heart, my eyes filled with tears of salt. My throat closed, and I whispered, "Oh yes! I love you."

# Siblings

## DOROTHY SCHULER

One day the woman realized that balding men do make better lovers.

So she went to the library to discover why: androgen, the hormone that causes "regression of scalp hair" and at the same time "growth of body hair" (she ran her mind across her lover's body, but had to stop; she was in the library) also increases a man's sexual desires and his "level of functioning."

The woman smiled secretly to herself as she pushed the encyclopedia back onto the shelf—and very surreptitiously caressed the books with her body, rubbing her breasts hard against the leather bindings.

The woman and her lover never discussed their relationship. He didn't know her last name or her phone number or where she lived. She wrote to him on delicately painted erotic Japanese cards with no return address on the envelope. The woman was in control.

She ran her hands down the sides of her body, stopped at her waist, stroked the soft curves of the hips. The body in the mirror had changed; tauter, it glowed under her touch. The woman cradled her breasts with her hands, missed her lover and imagined his hands playing with her nipples.

Steam seeped out the sides of the waffle iron as the lid closed. She watched it rise and dissipate in the crisp morning air and then went to the phone and called her lover.

"I thought of being in bed with you and I'm excited. I want

to feel you inside me. I want to lick you—all over your body."
Before he could respond, she softly hung up the receiver.

As she turned back to the kitchen she looked out the window, saw her husband and stopped to watch him water his garden.

"Hi," she said when he answered the phone. "Do you have time for lunch?"

"Go take off your underwear. Come to me just that way." Neither of them said goodbye, they just hung up.

She did what he said and left the office, and as she descended in the elevator with the men in their three-piece suits she blushed, hoping none of them could tell.

The drive to his studio was quick, all of five minutes, yet by the time she arrived her unprotected thighs were wet. The woman reached between her legs and coated her fingers with her own moisture. She licked them, amazed at her behavior, but excited by her taste.

The heavy, twelve-foot-long wooden bay door to his studio was open and she climbed up the three-foot ledge and walked in. He was waiting for her, naked, behind the door. Immediately, he slid it shut and, without even saying hello, began to kiss her.

He laughed when he tasted her mouth. Watching her face, he clasped her hand in his, reached under her skirt and guided her fingers, entwined with his own, deep inside her. He raised her fingers to his mouth and his to hers; together they tasted. Again he led their hands under her skirt and inside her.

Holding her that way, he walked the woman across the room to the couch. He extricated his fingers, unbuttoned her blouse and caressed her breasts, leaving a trace of her scent on them as he ran his hands up her throat and through her hair.

They made love, him naked, her still dressed, his arms grasping her close to him as if without her he could not exist. When they finished he undressed her and carried her to his bed and made love to her again, this time slowly, with less urgency.

When the hour was over the woman put on her clothes and went to the mirror to fix her makeup. She saw at once that her hair was different, fuller, shinier, and that her skin was smoother. She wondered if any of the men in the office would notice.

She turned off the hot water, felt the cool water running into the tub through her outstretched fingers and remembered her lover. He threaded his way around her thoughts as she soaped her daughter's body and squished the bubbles over the tender young skin, making her daughter laugh.

When the woman recalled taking a shower with her lover (their bodies glistening against each other as they made love, the steam enveloping them, water droplets clinging to her hair wet halfway down her back; he teasing her and watching as she played with herself in response, lathering her flesh and gliding her hands up and down the insides of her thighs and back and forth across her breasts) she was lifting her daughter out of the bath.

She tucked her child into bed and read her *Alice in Wonderland*.

The intensity of their lovemaking occasionally scared her; she thought she might become lost and never return. Sometimes the next day she would find a thumbprint on her thigh, a tender spot on her breast close to the nipple. Once both her breasts were covered with tiny bruises; she examined them carefully and counted them, thirteen in all.

It was her ritual to never visit him until the bruises faded, but as time went by, keeping to this self-imposed schedule became difficult. She sent away to a mail-order house for an herbal remedy purporting to make bruises heal faster. The potion worked and they faded in half the time.

His studio was their playground. They made love in every corner, on every surface, until the woman felt she knew his space as completely as his flesh.

She visualized one of his sculptures, "Siblings," the visual portrayal of incestuous desire, of words that cannot be spoken, acts that must be suppressed, emotions that must be controlled.

Two translucent marble forms, arms and bodies entwined, are lying side by side on a black marble bed. The larger figure is a woman; the other a man. The man caresses the woman's full, marble-veined breasts, pressing them together with his hands while he sucks on both of her nipples, his face nestled in her white flesh.

After she saw the piece, the woman always thought of her lover as her brother.

The woman woke to find her breast in her lover's mouth. She turned toward him and pulled his head closer into her body, his mouth taking more of her into him until she filled him completely. They had been lovemaking for hours, and now the sounds escaping them were quiet, in unison, whispers of insatiable desire, a hunger for each other that could never be satisfied.

When he came they were kissing, and he screamed into her mouth, his lips pressing hard against hers, sealing the sound within their bodies. It echoed back and forth between them.

Later, she got up, hating to let him slip from inside her,

and saw that they were covered with her blood. She washed herself and then gently and slowly cleansed his body.

She watched him water his grapevine. It grew in the central courtyard of a building in the smoggy downtown industrial area. The vine, planted many years before when the district was a vineyard, crawled up the scarred brick wall, two twining gnarled branches that spread and covered the lattice roof of the small courtyard. She was astonished that the plant continued to grow in the four-inch patch of undernourished city dirt.

The woman watched as her lover, little by little, poured water into the dirt patch; the vine slowly sucked it up. He tipped the pitcher and poured more water. The vine slowly sucked it up.

She wished that she were the vine, watered by her lover, patiently.

He filled the crystal glass with cognac, handed it to her and then lifted the bottle and spilled the sweet, thick liquor over her shoulders. It flowed across her voluptuous breasts, through the deep hollow between them, down the axis of her body, past her navel and into her pubic hair, leaving the trace of its course on her flesh.

She laughed and drained her glass with one swallow before reaching her arms out to him. He bent his head down to her cognac-soaked breasts, and as he licked and sucked the luscious liquid off her body the woman began to cry.

# Picasso

## MARY BETH CRAIN

There was something about Josef Forster that was never quite real. Something that transcended the obviousness of ordinary manhood. His sexual energy was frightening, almost suffocating.

He was a legendary concert pianist. I met him at a reception, one of those stale affairs that you try to slip into and out of as quickly as possible, like a bathtubful of tepid water. As a writer for a leading music magazine, I had attended the event purely out of duty, and after fifteen minutes of nondescript chitchat with nondescript chits, I was more than ready to flee. Suddenly, however, a laugh cut through the torpid air, a fabulous, ringing laugh that made every head in the room turn in its direction.

"I have just returned from Europe. England? God forbid! Why should I want to go to England? No, darling, I prefer the company of my native Austria. Why, when the Viennese were sitting very nicely at tables, eating with silverware and drinking proper wines, where were the British? Up in the trees, cracking nuts. . . ."

And Josef Forster entered the room like a long, sharp knife, about to cut the boredom to shreds.

He was very tall, six three or six four. Dressed in a perfectly tailored gray tweed suit, with a silk handkerchief peeping out of the breast pocket, he looked as though he had just stepped out of GQ. A cigar was balanced delicately in one hand; the other caressed the air with a series of flowing, unhurried gestures.

I felt a tightness in my chest, the gripping sensation one experiences upon realizing that the formless clay of one's everyday life is about to be molded into something significant. I could not take my eyes off of him, and neither could anyone else. The men were intrigued, delighted by his presence. But the women were completely helpless. The fact that he was, at that time, seventy-three years old was irrelevant; within five minutes every female in the room was veering toward him, exactly as a pile of quivering pins might be sucked up by a steel magnet. And through it all, Forster stood there languid and relaxed, flashing every now and again a dazzling smile that, like a massive generator, seemed to light up all of the faces around him.

I edged closer to him, and the nearer I got, the larger he became. He had the longest legs I'd ever seen, immaculately sheathed in pleated pants. A warm stream of excitement ran through me, a buzzing current that made me want to rub up against him like a cat or, better yet, to feel those long legs of his gripping mine.

At that moment, as he turned to look for someone, Forster glanced at me and I found myself frozen by two steel-gray eyes that, like the lenses of a camera, were semiclosed, impervious, opening only for a second to absorb everything about me.

He gave me the once-over. A flickering judgment, a mental disrobing. But he did this so smoothly, so deftly and with such elegance that while I felt stripped, revealed both physically and emotionally, I was not offended. And Forster smiled at this, ever so slightly, before moving across the room with his long, languid stride, in the direction of the person he'd been searching for.

I knew then that I had to have him. The age gap of forty-nine years was insignificant, a minor chasm easily bridged by

the invincible girders of charisma and desire. For the first time
in my life I was in the grip of raw sexual yearning, and the
fleeting click of Josef Forster's ocular shutter had thus recorded
the end of one chapter of my life and the beginning of another.

From a girl who lived in T-shirts and jeans, I metamorphosed
into a woman who began haunting dress racks, in search of
the sexiest attire I could find. I lost weight, got contacts,
experimented with lipsticks, eye shadows, perfumes. Somehow, instinctively, I knew the sorts of things Forster would
like, and always, before I chose a blouse, skirt or scent, I
conjured up the memory of his steel-gray eyes, washing over
me, registering approval.

And as I matured weekly, daily, things that had until now
been insignificant in my life became infused with eroticism.

I visited an art museum and saw a sculpture exhibit of nude
young women. Ordinarily I would have viewed the pieces
dispassionately, but now I saw them as Forster would have.
The small, firm breasts, the round behinds, the tantalizing
blandness of the virginal faces. I reached out and touched one
girl's bronze buttocks and the animal named arousal, frisky but
invisible, nipped me in my groin as I imagined that it was
Forster who was stroking my own cheeks with his long, delicate
hands.

I went down to the beach. This had always been a favorite
pastime, as I lived a block from the ocean. But now, as I
stretched out on the sand, I felt, instead of the sun, Forster's
warm hand, burning a slow path down my stomach, to the
insides of my thighs, stopping at last at my sex to penetrate
it with his experienced fingers, at first gently, then relentlessly.

And, as the waves crashed and subsided against the sand, I
closed my eyes and tried to imagine his penis inside of me,
pounding, exploding, retreating.

His penis. What was it like? I imagined it was as long as the rest of him, and as stately, but in truth I didn't care. I was in love with it whatever its shape or size. I was in love, in fact, with all of Forster—his legs, his ass, his wit, his charm, his paunch, his wrinkles... Was I mad? Did I really want to go to bed with my grandfather? Or was my infatuation merely an indication of simple good taste?

I had no idea, really. I knew only one thing: that I had to make Josef Forster love me back.

And so I got my editor's okay to interview Forster for a cover story.

I awoke early the morning of the interview, to spend as much time with my preparations as a bride on her wedding day. I luxuriated in a tubful of scented oil, chose my most smashing outfit, applied my mascara with the slow, deliberate strokes of an artist. I was prepared to seduce him, but I was also scared to death. Would he put down his cigar and take me in his arms? Or would he merely laugh? Or, worse, show me to the door?

By the time I arrived at his house, my nerves were on the verge of mutiny, and the shrill scream of the doorbell nearly gave me cardiac arrest. Several moments passed and I considered the possibility of bolting. And then the door opened, slowly, and Josef Forster stood there, looking breathtakingly suave in a pair of white Levi's and a blue silk monogrammed shirt.

"Come in, my dear." He held out his hand. His touch was polite, pleasant; he had, as one would expect, a large hand, within which mine was completely lost. It seemed odd to feel it so relaxed, and I had the sense that it was hiding its true identity. I had the sense, in other words, that Forster could break my hand off at the wrist in one squeeze, for the sinews were taut and the musculature was not that of a man of seventy-three.

"I love your shirt," I said. "Are all of your things monogrammed?"

Forster grinned down at me. "Everything, my dear. With the exception, of course, of my underwear, as I am never sure where I may leave it." He paused. "Have we met before?"

"Well, we didn't actually *meet*. I saw you, at the reception for Misha Behrman."

"Ah, yes." He looked down at me thoughtfully, sucking at his cigar, the scent of which permeated the room and was as sweet to me as the most exotic cologne.

"Your hair is shorter, is it not?"

"You remember that?"

"I never forget a woman. And you are thinner. Have you taken a lover?"

"Not one," I laughed. "Six."

"Ah!" He nodded approval. "This can have its advantages. But you must be careful not to exhaust yourself. I once had four ladies at one time, but then, I was young and could go for twenty years without sleep."

"And now?" I asked, shocked at my own boldness.

He chuckled, a rich, melodious sound that, like the scent of his cigar, filled every inch of the room.

"Now? My dear, now I cannot go for twenty *minutes* without sleep. I doze off in the middle of sentences..."

"Can you stay awake for our interview?"

"I shall try." He flashed one of his dazzling smiles. What made it so compelling, I noticed, was not mere seductive charm. It was also a smile of great sweetness, a combination of boyish mishievousness and kindly old age.

"Would you like a tour of my fortress?" he inquired. Before

I could answer, he was leading the way through a living room that might have been transplanted from Hapsburg Vienna with its antique furniture, bookshelves full of German volumes and dark oil paintings of Austrian landscapes. It was a strange room, I thought, virtually frozen in time. And yet beneath its old-fashioned exterior ran an unmistakable undercurrent of sensuality. The plush green velvet sofas beckoned, secure in the awesome silence that reigned throughout the house.

"These are original scores of the Brahms piano concerti," Forster was saying, in front of the bookcase. He pulled one off the shelf and stood there beside me, leafing through it. But as I bent over to look, I noticed that if I glanced sideways through the buttonholes of his shirt, I could see the forest of white hair on his chest.

"It's beautiful," I murmured.

"Would you like some coffee?" he said suddenly.

We went into the kitchen. This room had an odd sense of never having been lived in. The copper-bottomed pans, hanging all in order above the stove, were as shiny as if they'd never been used, and the gleaming aluminum counter top had not so much as a scratch. While the living room exuded a cozy languor, the kitchen seemed cool and crisp, but this was erotic to me as well. While Forster busied himself making coffee I envisioned myself naked, sitting atop the sparkling counter, which was shockingly cold against my flesh. Here, on this impersonal alloy, I was utterly submissive, a female steak that could be plopped, at any time, on the nearby chopping board. Before me stood Forster, smiling tenderly, sucking his cigar and drawing my legs up to reveal my wet, pleading lips.

"Mein Kleines," he murmured in thick, silky tones. "Mein Herzchen. Du bist so schön, so schön..."

And he bent down, gallantly, to kiss my hair, my mouth,

my breasts, my belly, as I thrashed blindly on the now steaming counter top and the pots and ladles watched, beaming, from the wall.

"Hey you!" Forster's voice, amused, brought me to and I realized that I'd been staring at the counter for a full minute. I blushed and suddenly, for the first time, Forster looked directly and intently into my eyes.

Did he know? Could he tell? But the moment, lightning-quick, was over. "Do you take milk?" he asked as he strode to the refrigerator.

He poured the coffee, meticulously, and took the tray into the living room. "Sit down," he said, motioning to the sofa. I hoped he would join me, but instead he sat down across from me in a large easy chair, his long legs looking incredibly youthful in the white Levi's.

"Where did you get those jeans?" I asked.

"Why?"

"Well, I've never seen a man your age wearing them, let alone looking good in them."

He laughed delightedly. "I bought them at Miller's Outpost, darling. It is marvelous, you know, up until ten years ago I could never walk into a store and buy a shirt, or a pair of pants."

"Why not?"

"Because of the *length*. My arms and legs were always oversized, in my generation, and in Europe, I was a giant. But after the war, in America, the young men grew like weeds. And the sizes have finally caught up with me."

"What did you do until then?"

"Oh, I had my own mannequins. In London, and Paris. And the most charming tailors..."

As he talked, he stretched his legs, opening them slightly. I began to ask him questions while glancing furtively at his crotch. The Levi's revealed a large bulge. Not an erection but an ample apparatus that lay there, as languid as Forster himself, waiting, it seemed, with catlike patience.

"Your face is red," Forster remarked. "Shall we go into the other room, where it is cooler?"

"N-no," I stammered.

"Where were we?"

"Your first U. S. concert tour. When was it?"

"Nineteen thirty-six . . . or was it '35?" He sighed. "Forgive me, my dear. I remember nothing anymore. But we can check on it."

He rose, walked over to the bookshelf and extracted a large volume. Then he came over to the couch and sat down beside me.

"My clippings, 1935 to 1937."

He opened the large leather-bound scrapbook. It had a musty smell. A magnificently sultry face looked up at me from the yellowing page. Josef Forster, aged twenty-four.

"My baby pictures," Josef chuckled.

"You were just my age."

"Well. And you are a baby, after all." He flipped through the pages, enjoying the little journey backward in time. I studied the photos of him, the wavy blond hair, sensuous mouth, heavily lidded eyes, slim physique.

"I can't decide whether I like you better then—or now," I said.

He laughed. "You are very sweet. Do you have an astigmatism?"

"I'm nearsighted."

"Ah! I have always had good luck with nearsighted women. Now—here we are. 'Josef Forster Arrives in New York.' Nineteen thirty-six, October."

Then his eye fell on another photo on the same page, of a

beautiful woman in an evening gown. "Maria Landauer!" he exclaimed.

"Who was she?"

"A marvelous singer. And a marvelous mistress."

I fought an irrational spasm of jealousy. "Yours?"

"Not only mine. She was valued throughout Europe. Ah, she was divine; she knew what she was doing. She had one perfume for her breasts, another for her armpits, another for her vagina. Ah yes, there are perfumes one can use there, special ones."

He turned to me, puffing slowly at his cigar. "You should buy one, to try out on your lovers."

"Where can I get it?" I asked.

He shrugged and turned the page. "That looks like Picasso!" I said.

"It is. We were good friends. He painted me once, in fact, but I told him it was a piece of shit. And he agreed! Ah, he was a devil . . . you know, when I saw him last, he was eighty-six and had a twenty-six-year-old wife on his arm. Of course, the world conceives of this as abnormal, but in reality it makes perfect sense."

"Why?" My heart was beating quickly.

"Older men are good for younger women. They cannot ejaculate every five minutes, you know; it takes considerably more time. And so the lovemaking is slower, more leisurely . . . Good God!" He glanced at his watch. "I had no idea the time had gone so quickly. We had better finish with your questions." And he rose and returned to his easy chair.

We spent an hour together, a marvelous, inimitable hour during which we bantered back and forth in a verbal fencing match that kept my arousal level at fever pitch. Every once in a while I would glance at my own watch, wishing desperately that the hands could be turned back. Finally Forster turned to me.

"It is getting late, my dear. Do you have all you need?"

No, I wanted to answer. I don't have you. But my courage failed me.

"I guess so," I said.

"Good." He rose and I followed him to the door, feeling as though I could not return to a world that didn't include him. He must have seen this in my face, for when I looked up at him to say goodbye, he reached out suddenly and touched my cheek.

"My girl," he chuckled. "My little girl."

My instincts finally overtook my intellect then, and I reached up and put my arms around him. Had I thought about it, I never would have dared to do it, as he seemed so huge, towering, formidable. But when I felt his body against mine, a great shock went through me. He was slim, frail, and his bones, which protruded at the elbows and shoulders, seemed brittle. Tears came to my eyes.

He looked down at me and the usually impervious gray eyes were pierced with sadness. Not understanding, I buried my face in his chest. His silk shirt was smooth and cool, and I wanted to tear it off of him. He trembled, and this gave me the courage to run my hands down his back, to his small, firm buttocks and at last around the front of him, where his long penis lay beneath his clothes and my hand, soft and silent.

Strangely, the fact that he had no erection did not bother me. On the contrary, I felt as tender toward his shy manhood as though it were my own sleeping child. But Forster pulled away from me and removed my hands from him, gently but firmly.

"You love an old man, my dear," he murmured.

"You're not old!" I sobbed, fiercely. "You're beautiful!"

"And you," he laughed gently, "are nearsighted." He walked to the door, opened it, and kissed me lightly on the forehead.

"Do not wear yourself out with your six lovers, darling," he smiled. "You must space them well."

I held him in my arms. The room was strange, alien; there was a small bed but no other furnishings, and I was blanketed in darkness. I was not sure where I was, and yet wherever I was, it seemed the right place, the only place to be, for his body was against mine.

"My darling," he murmured, as I reached down into his bathrobe.

"I love you, it's all right," I whispered, taking his huge balls into my hand and massaging them. They were soft and full, and the more I fondled them, the more excited I became. He moaned and his penis nuzzled its way into my hand. He was large, pulsing; I felt a tremor of amazed joy as I stroked the hard, violent flesh. My palm was hurting; his thrusts grew more demanding, his body heavier against me. And then he exploded in my hand with a strangled cry and I came myself, without having been touched...

I had this dream over five years ago, but it is still as vivid in my mind as the night I awoke from it, convinced that it had been more than mere illusion. For one thing, I had orgasmed in my sleep. But far more startling than this was the tingling sensation in my palm where I could still feel Josef Forster's sperm and where, when I looked down at it in the moonlight, a thin pool of moisture, transparent and warm, had settled.

# 1968

## SIGNE HAMMER

In the summer, New York has the sultriest air in the world. It smells of every age and variety of sweat: the musky odor from young men's armpits, the light tang from the backs and faces of girls on the subway, the resinous, locker-room brawl of stink from the workmen digging their trench.

It smells of fruit and vegetables: sharp citrus tang of oranges sliced and smashed and juiced for the throat; dizzying fumes from mounds of bruised and broken-skinned tomatoes, over-ripe plums and bananas and melons, thin-skinned grapes bursting in the sun.

It smells of smoke: little drifts of smoke from cuchifritos frying in iron pans set close to the earth over wood fires in Central Park; thick, pungent gusts pouring from shishkebabs grilling over charcoal on wagons in Times Square; marijuana smoke tantalizing the nose everywhere.

Musk, fruit, smoke, even the acid reek of garbage, the sudden dank-cold draft from an alley or open cellar, the bituminous stench of iron and steel and cement cooking all day in the sun, combine to release in the flesh fantasy and desire, as though the sheer incomprehensible quantity of smells overwhelms everyday decorum and the schooled self gives up, exhausted.

It is a slow walk across Eighth Street from Sixth Avenue to Tompkins Square Park. On the block between Broadway and Astor Place, I become aware of his back. It is bare, sweating slightly, the color of a ripe apricot. I loiter behind him across

the long series of intersections to Third Avenue, past the dingy
takeout place at Lafayette, past the subway and Cooper Union.
I am admiring his short, powerful forearms, the tender modesty
with which his shoulders curve into his biceps, the way his
buttocks, firm as ripe mangoes, move under his torn cut-offs.
His calves are high and round, with fine, springing hairs
bleached almost blond from the sun.

I catch up with him at an Italian ice cream stand. He is
buying lemon. I order lemon, too, and glance at him. His hair
and eyes are black, his face is a blend of Chinese and Hispanic.
His eyes are large and round but, astonishingly, manage also
to angle slightly upward at the outside corners. His nose is
thick and sensually curved at the nostril. He smells of fresh
sweat, sweetly tinged with aftershave. I imagine what his hair
would smell like if I put my face against it, gently. It is very
fine, with the matte-black sheen that comes from washing with
soap.

He turns and walks on and I follow, licking my lemon ice
from its little cup. He glances back and then slows by a step
until we are almost parallel, he strolling along next to the curb
and I next to the shopwindows, as if I were planning to stop
into a store. Across the sidewalk, we exchange little oblique
glances.

The lemon ice is cool and sharp on my tongue. The sun is
melting it quickly, and the juice runs down my chin and hands.
He licks around his mouth as far as his tongue can reach, like
a cat, then turns his inclined head as if to lick his shoulder, a
long, slow stroke on the curve of muscle, instead brings his
face up, looks full at me and grins. I grin back, and something
clicks into place between us. We are no longer two strangers
who happen to be walking in the same direction; we have
entered into a conspiracy of attraction.

At Avenue A we turn together into a little coffeeshop facing the park and take stools at the counter. He orders coffee, I order tea. Waiting for our orders, we flirt. I notice his eyebrows grow into little fans on the inside corners. The brows are thickly ridged in the middle, making him look very serious until he smiles. We are smiling a lot.

Teacups were designed for flirtation. The cup is brought tenderly toward the mouth, the lips open in a kiss shape to cover the rim gently, the eyelids rise so your eyes meet his in a smile just as the hot liquid meets your throat.

After a while, we slide off our stools, pay our checks and walk on together. We are moving toward my destination, because it is close, but we still have not spoken to each other. He has yielded his will to me, or to chance, and we are moving on a slow, eddying current of time.

At Sixth Street we walk up four flights; I am slightly ahead of him, conscious of his eyes on me. A little warmth grows in my vulva, a little tickling throb starts up, and time shifts, speeds up in anticipation.

The loft belongs to a friend of mine who deals only to people he knows. The sun pours in tall windows. On a low table a tray is spread with dark-brown cakes of hashish. We examine the different marks etched in the cakes and painted on the little bags in which they are sold. My friend shaves a few curls from a cake marked with a red horse's head and we smoke, and everything slows down again.

In the sweet, pungent smoke, the heat rises in my body, spreads to include the man who lounges next to me, his hand brushing my thigh. The back of my head floats, wide open; my legs and shoulders are relaxed, heavy. The hand by my thigh seems directly linked to the pulse in my vulva; I curve my body around the pulse and ride on it, circling outward and back with the sweet, stately pace of time. The sunlight shifts, deepens; minute, suspended points of dust turn gold.

Slowly, the pulse and the heat gather force inside me, and I sit up. So does he. The current between us has changed again, become active. I make my trade with my friend, money for hashish, and we leave.

Outside, it is late afternoon. The edges of things—buildings, leaves, cars—look slightly smudged in the humid air. We are both immediately damp, although we keep a little distance between our bodies as we turn west on Astor Place. The people who walk there dress to invent themselves; they wear purple robes and silver combat boots and long sweeps of hair and mustache; or baggy Zouave pants in many-colored stripes, with little flaps of cloth over their breasts. They walk high on sandals with immensely thick wedge soles; they are kings and queens in a kingdom of make-believe.

We walk among them, feeling their costumes a disguise for our own bodies. Occasionally, the backs of our hands touch, and we smile, both looking straight ahead, and sometimes we glance quickly at each other and smile again. We smile the secret, smug, delighted smiles of children who feel sure of their treat—chocolate cake, perhaps, with its thick fudge icing in one smooth slab over the moist, brown, velvet softness of the cake.

At Gem Spa we stop for egg creams, thick and sweet with just the faintest bluff, dry taste of seltzer around the edges. We stand at the little marble counter surrounded by magazines and paper-napkin dispensers and suck the dregs noisily through straws. The magazine teasers are all about sex. The cover photos are of women with pasties on their nipples and their legs spread wide, a round white sticker pasted over every crotch. Or they are of women draped in filmy lingerie, just the round of a breast and a high-shaven line of pubic hair peeping out. The round stickers draw the eye, each one a blank, a sanitary wasteland. The high-shaven pubic hair is like topiary, an illusion. We walk on without touching.

Astor Place becomes Eighth Street, and he takes the lead into the Eighth Street Bookstore and upstairs, to the art books on their big tables. He locates a book of Oriental erotic engravings.

In the Japanese section, the men all have huge purple cocks, the women achieve extraordinary positions and are displayed with the huge cocks partly inside them, while their faces remain smooth, expressionless, as if they were photographers' models posing for an underwear ad. The faces of the men are equally expressionless, but their eyebrows make them look fierce, determined. The women do not look at all surprised to find themselves in these positions; upside down, nearly standing on their heads or moving up on the monstrous cocks at a dead run, arms and legs frozen in a stylized frenzy.

I move on. In the Persian section, I stop at a picture in which six women disport themselves around a single man. He lies on his back in a sort of bathrobe, loosely belted, open down the front. Each woman has claimed an appendage; two loll by his hands, while his forefingers diddle their hot red vulvas; two more, their clitorises cunningly drawn, are served by his richly jeweled big toes. A fifth sprawls by his head so his tongue can caress her; the sixth lowers herself delicately, deliberately, onto his lively-looking little cock. I imagine a progression, from finger to toe to tongue and, finally, to the pièce-de-résistance. Afterward, the slow denouement of finger or toe again.

I look at this picture for a long time. The jeweled toes set the pulse in my vulva to throbbing again, while the living man leans into my shoulder. One arm steals around my ribs, a finger brushes my nipple, returns, caresses it through the thin T-shirt material. His big toe, innocent of jewels, strokes my instep.

When we leave the store, he keeps his arm around my waist. I lean into him. We fit. My hip, slightly higher than his, curves neatly into his waist; his shoulder tucks into my armpit; I curve my arm over his shoulder, around his back to his waist. His hair smells soft, slightly sweet around the sideburns. The skin of his cheek is faintly downy and golden, like the skin of a ripe apricot. The curve of his neck smells like musk.

We walk west like old lovers.

# PLAYFULNESS AND HUMOR

## *The Fifty-Minute Hour: Between the Minutes . . .*

*UNSIGNED*

In my office, a hot day, a talked-out therapist with too many patients, too many hours, days, indoors, in this hard chair. I long to stretch my legs, to wander into water not too cold, so that I can slowly, gently glide into the sea letting the water slide up my thighs. Greece. The Aegean. Oh, the water there. And A. Lying on white sand, our heavy straw bag filled with fruit leaning against the big rock. A breeze hardly felt floats the arms of my thin sundress from the crevasse on the rock where it hangs. The heat nauseates. I get up, naked, my breasts heavy with the heat, my nipples slightly burned, and walk, quiet so as not to wake him, toward the water. A quick bit of cold against my swollen ankles. My palms cup the blue water and dribble it into my snake-curl hair, down my back, on my belly. I go under slowly, am completely wet, completely cool. A laugh comes on and I cannot help but yell to the sleeping man. He stretches, unknowing of the heat, rippling waves of it making him look vague, lost in the sand, the red towel covering his buttocks. He rises, comes toward me, expressionless from sleep. He eases into the water. We swim together, he holds me in his arms, tickles my ear with his wet mustache. That couple walks toward us. That couple we've been watching watching us, our naked bodies curled in sleep in the sand, now

curled in the water. They are German and loud. They think
we are also German. I fake it easily. A conversation starts. A.
and I are still entwined, my hip resting against his knee, his
foot propped on a small rock underneath. From the shore, the
Germans in their green bathing suits tell us where to go in
town, what restaurants offer good fish. We understand almost
nothing of what they say. We nod and smile in response. A.
holds my breast under the water, fingers my nipple. I hold his
cock, a balance pole against the waves. He is erect. My nipples
are erect. His hand cups my crotch, his finger now inching
between my legs. I feel the water swirl in my open space. We
continue the charade conversation with the couple. My breathing becomes shallow, my insides well, open to him. I settle
myself on top of his cock, still making small German talk, my
upper body quiet, unmoved from the posture it held when the
couple first approached. A. and I pretend to bob up and down
with the waves, swirling our arms in mock play. I laugh at
something the woman says. A. touches my clit, hard as a
pebble. I bounce, he thrusts. Still the conversation. How can
this be happening... Our bodies jerk together, we come. We
burst out laughing and congratulate ourselves. We've done the
undoable again. But this time in front of people who are telling
us about where to get fish for dinner. And in another language.

A timid knock on my door. I start, stunned out of my reverie.
I am sweating. I notice that exactly three minutes have passed
since my last patient. It is time to talk about her mother again.
The door opens and closes. Mrs. T. sits down.

Mrs. T. begins to discuss tonight's dinner party. As usual,
her anxieties focus on how she wants to be seen, particularly
by the men. The green silk dress with the décolletage might
expose her desperation for attention. Her black velvet suit

might portray her as too somber; on the other hand, its simple elegance would have appeal in tonight's crowd. Always the same conflict between the overt and the subtle...

Between her heavy pauses, I think of last night. I, too, wear a black velvet suit. Too rushed to shower before dressing, I quickly sponge my underarms and crotch. Since I plan to have dinner with B. and nothing more, I don't let the smells beneath my clothing matter. I spray on some light perfume and slip into a lilac silk camisole. When the doorbell rings, I realize how late I am. B. will be annoyed. I slide the straight black skirt over stockingless legs and pull on the mauve suede shoes. I run downstairs to answer the door. As B. helps me with my suit jacket, I am conscious of the rings of sweat already encircling my underarms.

Small talk in the car. Both of us feel slightly awkward from our lack of contact over the last few weeks. B. drops his free hand between my thighs, comments on their ever-present softness. I can smell his cologne.

The restaurant is decorated in shades of mauve and gray. This is the first time either of us has been here. Over the white rose and flickering candle on our table, we look at each other, slowly and thoroughly, for the first time that night. Our hands move tentatively toward each other. His fingers stroke the underside of my wrist. I take his lean forearm in my hands and twist the skin slightly in opposite directions the way he likes. We stare at each other. The waiter stands by the table waiting...

Dinner is simple but elegantly served. The orange of the pureed carrots offsets the dark-green vegetables; a white truffle shimmers on top of the meat. Throughout the meal I am aware of the heat between my legs, the tension in my breasts. I slip my foot out of my shoe and lean into B.'s crotch with my big toe. At moments, I feel his cock twitch and arch against my foot. In response, he reaches under the table, pushes my skirt still higher on my legs and strokes the insides of my slightly open thighs.

With dinner over, we decide to explore the restaurant's elegant decor. We find ourselves in a candlelit alcove next to the rest rooms. The air feels hot in this corridor. B. leans against the wall and calmly surveys the color scheme, the rugs, the lamps. Again, I catch a sudden whiff of his cologne. Intoxicated by his smell, I kiss him full on the mouth. His tongue presses hard against mine, slides across my teeth, along my lower lip. Our mouths still together, I tug him playfully into the women's bathroom. He resists at first, saying, "What if someone sees us?" but allows himself to be pulled inside. Our mouths still locked, my hand cups his crotch. It protrudes in a hard knot. I draw him into one of the two stalls, close the door behind us and resume our kissing. We are laughing but ardent in our groping, caressing. B. stands with his back to the toilet, his hands under my camisole, pinching my nipples erect with wanting him. I push him gently down onto the closed seat. He slips his hands up my skirt, pushing his fingers between my legs into the wet of me. He sucks his fingers, then lets me smell and lick them. I unbuckle his belt and motion that he should let his pants drop. My skirt hiked to my waist, I straddle him. His hard cock goes easily into me. The camisole straps slip off my shoulders. He licks my nipples, plays with my clit. As I slowly bounce up and down on his cock, we both moan softly. Our breathing quickens in unison.

Someone enters the bathroom and opens the door of the other stall. The latch squeaks shut. The newcomer rustles her skirt and stockings, then urinates. I shove my open mouth against B.'s shoulder to muffle the low moans in my throat that threaten to build into screams. I whisper hoarsely that he's the best fuck in the world. In synchrony with our noises, our neighbor makes a pushing sound with her voice and farts loudly. As I twist and tremble on B.'s open thighs, I lose my balance and almost fall off his lap. B. lifts his legs off the floor so as not to be noticed underneath the half wall that separates the two stalls. I realize that my feet are pointing toward the back of the stall. If our neighbor looks down she will definitely know that something is awry, but I am too close to coming to change my position. As we push into one another, I can feel the top of B.'s cock thrust hard against the deepest part of my insides. We both come, and I slap my hand over B.'s mouth to silence his groans. Midcome, we hear the stranger leave her stall, wash her hands and do something by the mirror. We wait for what feels like an hour. When the bathroom is empty, we readjust our wrinkled clothes and laugh. We leave the bathroom, delighted at having pulled off another impossible fuck.

I catch myself and refocus on Mrs. T.'s dinner party. She says she regretted having chosen to wear the green dress with the décolletage.

"Oh, yes, Mrs. T., it's true: spontaneous actions can get us into trouble; perhaps indeed you should have given more thought before taking off with F. as though you had no responsibilities." On the other hand, I thought to myself, thank God for the ability to behave unplanfully. I could feel a smug, delighted smile pass through my eyes and rest for a moment on my mouth as I mused on last night's escapade.

C. picked me up outside my office at seven. Though I felt exhausted from a long day of work, just seeing C.'s broad-faced smile beaming through his car window enlivened me.

As I entered his old battered sports car that we loved so well
with its torn convertible top and the door that wouldn't open
from the inside, I was struck by how handsome he looked—
his dark complexion and well-cut curly hair contrasted against
a light shirt and cashmere navy sports coat; his jeans fit snugly
along his thighs and buttocks. C. kissed me quickly on each
eye, said how good it was to see me again, and zoomed us
off in the direction of downtown. Driving along, we carried
on an animated discussion on the possibilities that lay before
us—a movie after dinner or maybe going dancing. But since
we were both tired and had more work facing us at our re-
spective homes, we doubted the probability of either.

We arrived at the block where the restaurant was, parked
the car and leisurely strolled toward the entrance. Our arms
went naturally around each other's waist. I let my hand drop
to the curve of C.'s behind as we walked and felt each delicious
cheek move up and down inside his jeans. At the threshold of
the door, we disentangled our bodies and C. pushed me gently
ahead of him, quickly caressing my ass. The restaurant, though
small, was already humming with people. The vision of white
wine and steaming escargots at the next table perked my hunger
and I began to get into the evening with more energy. C. put
his hand firmly on my thigh and hid our two faces behind the
tall menu and kissed me. It was a long, delicious kiss, warm,
eager, familiar.

As always with C., dinner was delightful. We talked nonstop, our chatter punctuated by frequent laughter and sudden
meetings of our eyes. Our glances would lock for a few moments, making me feel weak-kneed, excited. I could feel C.'s
hand become clammy in mine. I knew he knew I knew. . . .
We both knew. But we'd already agreed that tonight could not
be the night: we had already decided to return to our separate

houses to complete work that needed to be done by the next day. A little tipsy from the wine, we stumbled out of the restaurant and into the dark city street. Having vetoed the movie—we'd spent too much time at dinner and it was already late—we decided to drive to the Village and poke around before going our own ways.

When we passed a shop selling pornographic literature, I stopped in my tracks, peered inside and hesitantly asked C. if he'd mind going into the shop with me. Though I'd always been curious about these places, I'd never dared go in one. As we entered the small, overstuffed, poorly lit shop, I suddenly felt shy and self-conscious—what if someone I knew walked in—what if one of my patients saw me. . . . Soon, however, I lost my nervousness and, hand in hand with C., began to explore some of the pictures of men and women in every position imaginable. Cocks were huge, vaginas juicy and dripping with come, breasts gorgeous with nipples so red they looked raw. But aside from the pictures of women with animals, it was the ordinariness of the poses that struck me. I had expected to stumble upon something bizarre, something I'd never thought of, something wonderfully unique. Instead here were photographs of well-endowed men and women simply fucking in all the various but regular ways. I was made aware not only of how limited human sexuality is but of how common my own experiences were. We both acknowledged feeling disappointed, unenlightened and sadly unaffected.

Once by the car again, C. put his arms around me and we kissed long and hard. Though I was slightly surprised, I found myself responding immediately. Our tongues met and intertwined; C.'s hands glided softly over my breasts, his thighs pushing my back against the car door. When we heard a group of people walking toward us, we scrambled into the car—one behind the other—through the passenger door. Our bodies almost glued together, C. continued fondling my breasts, squeezing my excited nipples and kissing my neck. I felt his cock bulge beneath his pants. Simultaneously we became aware of the late hour and the total visibility of our car. Reluctantly but laughingly, C. drove us toward the street where my car was waiting. We both agreed that perhaps the porno shop had affected us a little in spite of our initial disappointment.

In spite of our resolve to end the evening immediately, we continued touching each other while C. drove. The tops of my thighs were wet with excitement; I wanted much more. Besides the creaking of the loose doors and half-coiled springs underneath the seats, the only noise in the car was the sound of our breathing and the rustling of our clothing underneath our caresses. I felt as if I was going to jump out of my skin with wanting C. But getting what I wanted, no, needed, seemed impossible. Everything conspired against us—the late hour, the tiny, uncomfortable car, our plan to end the night at our separate houses.

Yet by Fifth Avenue, we'd managed to get totally out of control. I'd unzipped C.'s jeans and was fondling his hard penis while he unhooked my bra and softly twisted my exposed nipples between the fingers of his free hand. He pulled over to the side of the busy, extremely well lighted street. Without a comment I squeezed myself onto the tiny floor and took his cock in my mouth. C. protested at first, reminding me of where we were—only on one of the busiest streets of New York—but soon he began moaning and whispering my name. Though I was aware that scores of cars were streaming by us and that we were parked so illegally that not getting caught would be a miracle, practical issues just didn't matter much. C. lay on the seat with his long legs crumpled against the window while he stroked my wet clit with his finger; I continued to lie curled on the two and one half feet of dirty floor on the passenger side hanging on to the stick shift for stability while sucking on his cock. With an energetic thrust, C. came, pushing the back of my head sharply against the dashboard. Now wedged impossibly underneath the steering wheel, I, too, came. Spent and exhausted, bruised, stiff, and very wrinkled, we slowly straightened out our folded bodies and crumpled clothes and lay against each other, chuckling.

The windows were too steamed up to see the approaching policeman. But there he was, knocking on the window, inquiring as to exactly why we'd stopped on this particularly dangerous spot at eleven o'clock at night. We explained something about having to look up a street on a map, assuring him that we were just about to leave. I could just see tomorrow's headlines: "Psychotherapist arrested for sucking off journalist on Fifth Ave."

So much for an uneventful, weeknight evening. So much for my cautioning Mrs. T. about the dangers of spontaneity while I sat there smiling inside and impatiently awaiting the next uneventful night with C.

# How I Spent
# My Summer Vacation

## UNSIGNED

The plane lifted off from the runway. Tons of plastic, pistons, passengers and passports all roaring toward Paris. For what? Tourists returning home sporting Disney World bags, New Yorkers clutching Berlitz phrase books memorizing the directions to the bathroom in the Louvre, business travelers reciting the litany of bottom-line prices for cement firms or studying the exchange rate, and me. I was fleeing the New York City summer in the throes of final agony.

Too many lovers. Too many choices. I had left my job to take a summer off to "think." Instead I had taken the summer off to "fuck." The solace was somehow not the same. August nights were longer and the position of the stars changed. The coming of fall vegetables told me summer was getting long in the tooth. I didn't have much time left to do what I had planned.

My deus ex machina had come in the shape of an old college friend. A rich Yalie who had dropped out junior year to pursue the pleasure of pastels in the South of France. She nearly tripped over me as I lay on the beach in East Hampton pondering the diminishing summer and tide. Her straw hat, à la Monet, had obscured her vision. Doubtless she was composing the perfect Eastern still life to take back with her to Belmont, France.

We exchanged the vital statistics of the last four years and she said, "You must come for a visit." Her garret was an old *presbytère* and it sat high on a hill between two valleys. It had become, she said proudly, "sort of a haven for women who are

looking about." She was going back in a week. I was welcome
to visit. I took her number in New York and said I'd mull it
over.

I called her bluff Monday afternoon. I knew her type. All
that breeding. It forces them to make offers you aren't supposed
to accept. She couldn't back down. I needed a place to go to
write, to think, to escape the parade of pricks that had passed
through my legs in the past three months.

So there I was, Pan Am to Paris. One night of eating snails,
a day at Beaubourg and then the early train from Gare St.-
Lazare to Bretenoux by way of Brive. My friend had given me
the time and track and after a six-hour ride through fairy-tale
farms and fields I would land and her driver would meet me.
Dinner would be waiting.

Belmont sits smack on a hill that rises up between St.-Ceré
and Bretenoux in southern France. The region is known for its
pâté, caves, cows and wine. The *presbytère*, built in 1608, was
a large walled complex. Whitewashed stone walls, choir loft,
former altar cloths for curtains, big wooden beds, wide slatted
floors, marble tubs and fireplaces in every room. It was beautiful. Peaceful. A miracle.

Two other women were in residence, Mary a photographer
from Africa and another painter named Zoë from Paris. The
five of us ate dinner together every night to compare work
and adventures. I spent the days traipsing through the countryside by bike eating the plums, blackberries, walnuts, figs
and apples that graced the roadway. I wrote in the evenings,
ate, walked under the stars and slept.

The fire between my legs cooled. I slept with no men. They
had left my mind. The hot dreams that plagued me in New
York subsided. My cunt no longer woke me throbbing in midnight orgasm. In three days I stopped dreaming of hot kisses
or anal sex on the floor with a tall blond. After three weeks I

was content to be a nature nun.

My time in heaven drew to a close. I promised to meet two gay men friends. They were both artists and were showing at the Biennale. When I mentioned my spur-of-the-moment trip to Europe they cajoled me into joining them in Venice. The watchword for my itinerary was "Why not?"

I awoke abruptly on the morning of my departure. My night had been torn by dreams. The tall blond had returned and he stood at the side of my high wooden bed. He parted the curtains and pulled back my covers. He entered my cocoon. I was motionless. Pinned to the bed by the arms of Morphée and the reveries into which the God of Sleep had dragged me.

He pushed my white cotton gown up over my breasts and his long flat fingers traced the line of muscle that ran down my stomach and into my tangle of black pubic hair. We wore no clothes in our walled paradise and my skin was brown and the tiny cilia hairs on my belly and arms glistened golden. Almost as golden as the man whose fingers trotted up and down my body.

Down my thighs, up the insides just to where the cunt lips open and then back down again. Up my sides to my berry tits and browner nipples. He stopped and took them between his fingers and rolled them tight like the final stages in rolling a joint. Back and forth. I felt him stare down at me with his perfect ice-blues burning through my eyelids, which were frozen shut. He was bending toward me. I felt the pressure of his weight on my breasts and his hot breath spread a circle of heat first on my chest and then focused smaller and smaller till it hovered at my lips. A hummingbird with wings and heart at a febrile pitch unwilling to land. He brushed my lips. I stirred and he came back and nested in the soft inner reaches of my mouth. Cautious at first and then tonguing and searching. I was kissing back. Still unable to move—to touch the down on the back of his neck or to draw him into me further. He was so gentle in my mouth yet the pressure of his hands increased. He inched down from my mouth to my chin, chin to neck to sucking ears, and I knew where this meal would end. Honey head bobbing back and forth across my shoulders. Over my breasts sucking on the rock-hard nipples and passing his huge hands up and down my stomach. I tried to wake, to participate, to touch his head, but my arms were pinned beneath my head. I could not budge. He moved to my inner thighs and kissed so softly—wings against my flesh. My blond, my tease, then stood. I felt the circle of heat leave me to be replaced by the layers of linen and wool. He closed the curtain tightly around the bed and left.

I didn't wake from this dream. In the morning I was so goddamned hot. My calm, celibate core was shattered. The train arrived and I was off for Brive, en route to Nice. I sat facing a young boy. Perhaps he was sixteen. He kept staring at me and then down at the floor. He had a hard-on that grew during the trip. I knew I had "it" back again. That certain intangible something that I get, like being in heat. Once it starts seeping out of me men are attracted in droves. It is my core lusting after them. I have the smell and air of accessibility. Damn that blond for stirring all this up! Just when I thought I had capped it so snugly.

We stopped. The boy and I parted as I changed trains. Sunset sent shafts of gray and pink light into the big open-frame station. I paced up and down the track eyeing the travelers and scanning schedules. A conductor spotted my constant time-and-track checks and asked my destination. Yes, that train would be arriving on this track momentarily.

It did. And as I gathered my bags and new baskets and prepared to lug myself on board the same conductor came up behind me to help. "*À droit,*" he said. All the other passengers

were going left. I followed him right into an empty compartment. He set my bag down in the rack and turned on my
reading light. *"Bonsoir,"* he said and left.

He wasn't marvelous. He was dark and pouty and stocky.
He had shiny black button eyes. He was much like a stuffed
bear. I thought about what had just passed. It was my imagination. He was helpful. I was pretty and had *"un accent amér-
icain."* Some Frenchmen loved that. I tried to lose myself in
Proust, but it was too cerebral. I keep leaving Combray for
my covers in Belmont and my dream deferred.

Rolling and rocking the train moved south. I began to feel
sleepy. I switched off the main light leaving only the tiny tubes
illuminating the window edge. I pushed my nose to the glass
and looked out into the night. Nothing. No city lights. Blackness.

The door slid open and there stood the teddy-bear conductor. He sat and we began boring, limited French conversation. Had my French been better I might not have let him
kiss me. At least not so soon. He kissed me hard and Proust
fell to the floor. I contemplated for a moment whether I would
continue this or not. We had only one hour before we landed
in Toulouse. There would be no connections, no morning
coffee or conversation, and that tall blond had provided such
great foreplay for his opposite to consummate. We continued
kissing and his hands moved to my breasts. He sighed and
exclaimed and buried his nose and hands. *"Quelle poitrine formidable."* Such a soft mouth. He loved my body—and my hands
moved down under his jacket past the tickets to his skin. Up
and down his back while he moaned and pushed my hands
down to his cock. I rubbed him and he bit at my neck and
kissed softly into my ear whispering all wonderful and all hot
in French.

He stood and locked the door. He moved back toward me,

unbuttoning his pants, and in the half light I saw the head of his cock peep out from the top of his shorts. A drip of semen glistened. I lay back at first and let him take me. Let him kiss me and remove my shirt, my bra and sink into my tits. Groaning and purring every time his lips touched the skin or were enfolded by my large breasts. He kissed down my gut and stopped. My hands were inside his pants and wrapped around his prick. I stopped. We fumbled to stand. We were tangled in clothes and extremities. Finally we stood naked, two strangers in a speeding train. He came at me and returned his tongue to my mouth. No quest, just sucking, and his hands moved up and down me, fingering my breasts, cupping them, weighing them, and then he sunk to his knees. I fell back on the seat and he dove deep between my legs. I was dripping and he pushed back the edges and went for the juicy soft center. He never stopped licking and probing as he climbed onto the seat, rotating his body so that his cock came to rest in my mouth. I returned his sucking motions until I felt my cunt begin to contract and a hot flush spread from my toes to my cheeks. *"Plus vite,"* I said and he poured power till a hollow echo formed in my ears. I gasped and the train roared. My ears and cunt exploded. He was pleased. *"Tu es contente."* I could only purr and beckon him up to me.

As he stood I pulled him down so that his cock was between my breasts. He was still spit-wet and slipped easily back and forth as I pressed my breasts together tight around him. His head rolled side to side and he braced himself on my shoulders and pumped into my flesh. The train tore on and I felt sweet ripples come up through me as my body rocked on the leather seat. He stiffened and his weight fell onto my arms. He was crooning for more and then silence as he shot hot between my breasts, on my chest and under my chin. *"Tu es formidable. Je jouis."*

We didn't kiss or hold to each other. We were strangers. He found a handkerchief and wiped me dry. I told him I felt like a child being cleaned up—a very beautiful child. *"Une très belle enfant,"* he added and kissed my forehead. He went off to dock the train and I went to wash off in the tiny metal sink. My hair stuck to my neck and my cunt still streamed. I think his name was Jacques.

On time in Toulouse, I smiled as I left the train. It was quite an adventure and a great vindication of my hot night dream. My connecting train was ready and waiting. I found my *couchette* and snuggled into the sheet/blanket envelope. The compartment was empty. Strange because usually there are three to five others all rolled and stuffed. I lay on the edge of sleep and stayed there as the train pulled out bound for sparkling southern shores. Soon another conductor came in, looked at my ticket and began with earnest eyes to flirt and propose. I couldn't believe it. He was blond and mustachioed with blasting yellow-brown eyes. "No more," I thought. *No!* And I made it clear that I wanted sleep—only sleep—and he left. My God, three weeks of celibacy had left bundles of sexual energy creeping out everywhere.

I blinked in sleep and woke up to cold coffee and the rocky coast. I had to get to that beach. At Nice I grabbed my duffle and shuffled off.

I found a small room, cheap with breakfast and only a hop to the beach. With basket in hand, Proust and peaches in basket, I set off for the shore. The pebbles seemed to nestle into all the nooks and crannies of my back, filling in the missing links and massaging me. The sun baked my front. I lay cheek-to-jowl with other topless bathers. The languages were French, German, Italian and English.

Three young English speakers, two men and a woman, plopped down on the minispace left. The subway at rush hour was good preparation for this beach scene. Harsh twangy tones told me these were no main Island Brits; Australians perhaps. It was Sydney, to be exact, and the unattached man began conversation. "You speak English." "Yes, I think I still can," I returned. "Usually you don't see Americans topless on the beaches; it's a sure tip-off as to who they are. Why are you?"

"It's a disguise!" I snapped. He laughed. He was very pretty. Truly pretty with shoulder-length blond ringlets and angular features. About six feet tall, a bricklayer and surfer with attenuated muscles and skin so thin and fine and tan that it looked as if it had been chosen from a bookbinder's secret cache of Moroccan calf. Within this setting his eyes shone a pastiche of blues. Little chips of shell broken from robins' eggs and melted onto a hot marble. He was beautiful.

We compared itineraries. He was leaving for Rome that night. "Why not leave in the morning?" I asked. The *couchettes* were all saved and since he was traveling with his brother and sister-in-law they had to stay together.

By midday we wanted off the beach so we strolled back to my hotel propelled by my offer of a joint. We both tried to saunter into the hotel but the hawk at the door admonished me. *"Mademoiselle, c'est une chambre pour une personne. Vous!"* We tried to convince her, but the French despite the romantic marketing are hard-bitten. I went up, got the joint and returned to him waiting in the doorway.

Long deep drags of smoke filled my lungs and began to disengage my sense of real time. We smoked and walked. He had checked out of his hotel so we had the streets and beach. Leaning against buildings we kissed and pushed our pelvises into each other. I fingered his curls and licked some salt from his neck. We drank wine and ate raspberry sherbet on the beach. I was content not to force this moment to culmination. A little light romance after last night's accelerated crisis.

Train time. We walked to the station like two young lovers.
He was leaving for the war. I would stay and wait an hour or
two before finding someone else. Mad, deep kissing, excited
applause from the crowd. I blushed and he boarded the train
for Roma. I think his name was Alister.

Darkness was full and the town had become quite urban-
looking. Neon blasting in among arched passages, movies,
bars, oysters and perfume for sale. After a long walk through
town back home by way of the boardwalk and the ocean I was
ready for a night alone. Tomorrow I would be in Venice.

Back on the train and resettled by the window with Proust.
Blue, gray rock coves soon gave way to an endless dry yellow
landscape. Fields and factories alternated in my windows and
I was anesthetized by the images that moved past. At sunset
the most incredible sight began to appear. The yellow land
disappeared into gray water. We passed the first Venice station
and I readied my bags by the door. Boats of all sorts sprung
up on the water that surrounded the train and I knew we had
arrived. The sun sunk into the water and I thought I heard
that red ball hiss as it dipped behind the horizon spreading an
incandescent glow. I boarded a water taxi; it became my lover
taking me by the hand to where I had never been.

The boat followed the glow and the city spread out the
sparkles, the tinsel of night, and when I landed on the dock
Venice was in evening clothes. I was in jeans and dirty. I ogled
the diamonds of San Marco and pressed my nose to the elegance. I twirled around the square a solitary waltzer in a lu-
minescent music box.

Venice by day was less magical but full of sights and my
two friends had set up parties, openings and shows. Of course
interspersed in all this there was food. After a few days of
uneventful sightseeing I met my friends for breakfast at the
*pensione*. "Now, what are the big plans for the final night, fellas?"

I quipped. There was a dinner party being thrown at the villa of some Venetian art dealer. It sounded boring and organized. "Maybe I'll go off on my own. See if I strike it rich." "Oh no, we said we'd bring you. We need a woman. Besides, our host is incredibly handsome, rich, young and crazy." "What time is dinner?" They knew how to get me.

I fixed up my package just fine. White linen blouse and turquoise silk skirt, pearls, open sandals, hot lipstick and new perfume. The boys thought I looked great and with one on each arm we took off for the Grand Canal.

Immense, square and stone, the villa was impressive—even from outside. The doorman ushered us to the butler, who moved us upstairs, where the door was opened by our host. My cunt and jaw dropped at the same time. Standing there was a tall, lean, smiling Jean-Paul Belmondo with copper hair, a spray of freckles, shining teeth, teeming huge brown pools for eyes and hands so big and strong that I saw mine disappear up to the elbow when he shook it.

We were immediately drawn to each other; moths to a funeral pyre. I wanted immediate immolation, but he had to be the good host. Drinks for all in the most beautiful Murano crystal. The art was mind-boggling. I swear the True Cross and St. Peter's chalice were behind glass in the living room. Everything else sure was. Very classy. And he was amazingly insouciant. Dressed in faded Levi's, a custom-made Brooks Brothers striped blue oxford shirt, loafers, no socks and a $6,000 Rolex watch. A European preppy. I was in heaven. I talked to all the guests, using my best school Italian. I found out that at twelve we would go for a small dinner. The last supper in Venice.

The restaurant was right around the corner and he was well known there. Table and wine waiting, I managed to be seated so that only one person separated us. That person would be scorched by middinner by the heat of the sizzling conversation that passed between us.

Course after course paraded by and each one was saluted by a different wine. We were getting very drunk. Our host led the way. The roast was presented and he rose to carve. He was lousy and I chided him. "No finesse." With great ceremony he handed me the tools. I stood. Immaculate, pressed and shining, I moved to the head of the table and deliberately and brazenly sliced all the meat from the bones. It was a fabulous flirt.

Dinner moved to dessert, the formal structure broke down, guests milled around and he moved to the bar to choose aperitifs. I followed. I was so fucking hot in body and mind. I needed to go outside. I stopped at the bar to take a sip from his glass. "Good choice," I said and headed straight for the door. He followed me.

I braced myself on the wall by the canal and he sat next to me. I took his face in my hand and turned it toward me. I kissed him. He came back at me like an explosion. Like one of those funny trumpet-shaped yellow flowers that shoot seeds in summer if you so much as brush by it. They wait by the side of a path and entice you to touch and then they pop curly green tongues. He lifted me off the wall and, kissing me, he carried me into the alley next to the restaurant. I had never been with someone so strong, so crazed. "Sono caldo tremendiso," he muttered and we sweat our shirts through in a minute. Biting, clawing, his hands under my arms, my feet never touching the ground. "I am the host. I must go back in," he stammered. "Okay, let's go. Don't worry." I tried to kiss him softly but every touch drove him crazy. I wrestled myself from his clutches to the ground and tried to rearrange my sartorial image. Linen and silk wrinkle like hell. What the fuck; it was worth it. Give the boys a good giggle.

We returned. He sheepish, me triumphant. We finished dinner and headed back to the villa for more drinks. I was turning into a canal; I was so full of liquid. He was really bonkers, so frantic. It was wonderful. I came into the kitchen to assist; the butler was off. He grabbed me and those full movie star lips wrapped around me and we kissed and sunk back into one another. A shuffle from across the room disturbed our embrace. One of his friends setting out lines of coke, sorting the white powders into neat little regiments. Soldiers for review and inhalation. One-two, one-two and we had done them all. Now they would fire their guns inside our heads and into our blood. We kissed again as the rails raced to our brains.

Guests were leaving and my friends eyed me. Was I staying? "Oh yes," I said innocently. "We are going out for a ride in the speedboat." They tramped off into the night to catch a water taxi, but not before warning me, "The train to Paris is at noon!" The host no longer had guests to occupy him and we turned to each other. "Oh yes, the boat ride, as I promised," he said with the most wonderful, rich Italian accent. The doorman brought the low, long speeder around to the waterside door and we got in. He zoomed off, careening through the canals at breakneck speed. He turned to me. "Can you drive?" "Sure!" I retorted. I had never piloted a boat in my life, but he was very drunk, I was not, and I thought, "Shit! American girls can do anything." I trusted me more than I did him. We exchanged places and he began to coach me and kiss me and grab around me. "Watch out, don't hit one of those things; they are very heavy," he teased. I had the throttle full out and we bashed and bumped our way out of Venice. "Where are we going? Just thought I'd ask."

Like Count Dracula he growled, "To the sea." My heart was pounding, doing push-ups, sit-ups, curls, all at once.

He reached over and pulled back the throttle. The boat

went still in the water. We had laughed and talked and the engine had roared the whole way out. Now everything went silent. We hesitated for a second before devouring each other. His open mouth engulfed my face in much the same way as his hand had taken mine when the evening was young. We groped and kissed and grasped at each other. It was desperate and violent. We had hardly begun. Clothes began to fly around the boat. He arranged the cushions so that the floor was covered. There were enough to pad a space for even all six feet three of him.

He took off his pants. He had on those tiny bikini pants that you would think cliché Italians should wear. They do. His cock was gigantic. He bit me hard, shoved me to the floor and joined me. I could squeeze him, hug him, sink into him as hard as I wanted and he came back kissing, running his thick fingers down my spine, under my ass and between my legs. Teasing up and down my legs, resting inside my cunt for a moment, touring the folds and then jogging down to my knee. I was wriggling. There had been hours of foreplay and I wanted him, all of him, inside me.

The boat rocked beneath us and I split farther with every thrust and roll. He stood up and lifted me onto his hard partner, much the way you'd hoist a child onto a horse. Snug and secure we swayed ever so gently. Feeling the pitch of the boat and the message of my cunt, he steered us both so perfectly. He wedged his fingers down between my legs and rubbed deliberately on my clit. Pressure around and release and pressure as he held me with one hand beneath my bottom. I had ceased to be amazed at his Herculean quality. I was lost to the purple haze that began to enshroud me. The color came on me lightly at first and then clamped its hue and scent to my nose and mouth while my cunt flashed ringlets of electricity across my corpus. I could take no more. *"Vieni!"* I screamed into the clear star cover and he came as my purple pulse caused my cunt to bear down on that great huge cock. We were competing for contractions and throbbed at each other as his shot seeped down my spine.

Exhausted, we collapsed. Moonlight poured down and warmed us. Our sweat began to dry in the cool breeze as we fished our clothes off the boat bottom. I was in the stars, on Mars, or in heaven. Excited by this living fairy tale. The prince took me in his arms, folded me so tight and sighed.

"Can you drive us back? I will show you the way."

Dappled heaven light caught the silver trim and shot sparks into my sleepy, sleepy eyes. I drove carefully. My copilot hugged me and threw my hands up in the air over my head, grasping them and chanting, "The best driver on the Grand Canal. The best, the best." I was.

Even though I was the best driver the crazy Venice police still stopped us three times on the trip back. "It is because you are beautiful and they want to talk to you. The police love beautiful women late at night. So do I." He kissed the back of my neck.

Home safe. It took me two tries to dock the damn boat, but I persisted. One hand yanked me up out of the boat and into the bedroom.

The bedroom was on the top floor, glass-covered, high above the city of Venice. Red roofs, gray water, long low boat horns and marble church tops were the palette with which the room was decorated. Only all of Venice, a huge bed and a small table. On the table were a plate of figs and peaches and some mineral water. "These are the last of the season," he said. "We should eat them all."

He broke open a purple fig. The leather skin split to reveal a mélange of crimson, rose and salmon—all folded and ringed with seeds. The soft center pushed up and away with the

pressure of his two thumbs. He moved the delicacy toward
me. I tilted my head back and let it all in. Running it around
my gums, to the back of my tongue before swallowing. In
Italian the slang for vagina is fig. The metaphor was not lost.

We sat naked, eating the ripest fruit, dripping juices of all
sorts and talking as though we had been together for eons. In
other galaxies we had laughed about our fathers, or procras-
tination, the fear of failure, the love of the ocean, the exaltation
and paralysis of choice. I wanted to fly out the door directly
to the moon to stop its flight across the sky. To arrest time
and spend a year with those figs and that man as fresh and
ripe as they were.

We lay back in each other's arms to sleep, but as soon as
breast hit hard chest the restless night began again. The kisses
were deeper now and full of sighs and sweetness. The urgency
had been exorcised in the ritual of the sea and now we tongued
and cooed. He slid down my body kissing every part; we
giggled. I tapped my fingers on his freckles and rolled in
ecstasy. "Just one more most perfect fig," he said.

His thumb and forefingers opened my cunt and held back
the lips the same way he had offered me the first morning's
fig. Then my mind went blank as the oxygen was sucked away
from me by his huge soft mouth. No first licks, no touches.
Just his full wet inner lips locked onto mine. Mouth to cunt
he sucked every fold, the standing ridges, the helpless clit, all
into his mouth at once. He rolled and kissed and swayed and
then placed his hands under my ass to deliver the meal. Short
blasts of orgasm came out of me. Sparks and light like a summer
storm. My lights flashed on and off. My ears throbbed a hot,
sick sensation. He felt every jolt. I sensed his electrocution.

He released his suction hold and moved his tongue around
my cunt wildly; a silver disk shot from a pinball machine. Up
through the mazes, hitting all the stops, ringing the bells and

holding that damn machine, shaking it so that the ball tours and hits, again and again. The clanging, the ringing, the jingling, were almost more than I could bear. He finished the game by running his finger up and down my cunt; sucking and kissing violently. At the last minute he put his fingers up my cunt and into my asshole. The gong hit. The stars fell from the sky and as I opened my mouth to scream he stuffed the heel of his other hand between my teeth.

I wrapped into a ball and he tucked himself into the edges. There were very few hours left for sleep.

Bright morning came with *caffè latte* and brioches on the table where the figs had been. We gazed at each other with big moon eyes, ate, showered and dressed. "We must keep in touch," he said as we parted at the Grand Canal. I know his name was Vittorio!

My friends were at "our table" for morning coffee. Was I a ghost? They looked at me as if I had walked across the Grand Canal buoyed by some mystical power.

"We didn't think you'd make the train to Paris; as a matter of fact I had doubts we'd ever see you in New York City again."

"He had to go to Milano for business, I have to meet people in Paris. Hey, you guys, it's late. Grab your bags."

The vaporetto and Venice in blazing, relentless day was less kind than my gentle arrival. *Fable finito*, I was bound for Paris and another Pan Am jet.

# Truckin'

## BROOKE NEWMAN

As I approached the freeway I was thinking only of my testimonial and actual will. I don't usually think about my will—I am not terminally ill or particularly conscious about dying, though freeway driving can be hazardous—but today I had to consider it since I was on my way to my attorney's office to have the thing done properly. Now, I like driving and I like cars and I especially like trucks, so driving for me is a pleasure rather than an irritant and I usually like moving on from here to there in my four-wheel-drive, extended wheel-based CJ 7 Golden Eagle Jeep. Mine is the Jeep that has an eagle spread-winged on the hood, mine is the eight-cylinder Jeep that has more pickup climbing a hill than almost any typical American or foreign car on the road. Actually it would be safe to say that I love my Jeep and that we do well together; woman and car. I don't get absurdly involved with my car; at least I don't believe I do, though I may anthropomorphize a bit here and there. I feel, let's say, just lovingly toward my auto.

In any event, I was entering the freeway, thinking about my beneficiaries and how they would react to receiving bits of my life after I was gone and what my attorney would think of my generosity and goodwill when a semi pulled alongside the Jeep and, instead of passing, hung in there side by side at my speed. This semi was an eighteen-wheeler with shiny chromed doors, a stark black hood, chromed bumper, a long, long, long flatbed base that was not in the least rusted out (unusual for a semi), immense tires (each the height of my side-view mirror) and a red-and-gold decal on the door which said "Jack Driven," and beneath that a picture of two red cardinals facing each other. I figured that either Jack, who was obviously the owner-driver of the truck, transported birds across the country or that he had a thing for cardinals or he was a baseball fanatic from St. Louis. Whatever the case, Jack's truck was one hell of a fine semi. Now, looking over at Jack Driven's truck, I could only see his truck, I couldn't see Jack, and I wondered if he had seen me. Why else were we climbing the freeway grade together and neck and neck exceeding the speed limit? Unless he just liked Golden Eagles, I figured Jack had seen me as I entered the freeway. I actually do look hot behind the wheel: long flowing blond hair attracts truckers. And as Jack could no more push up that hill as fast as I than a turtle could outtrot a gazelle, I slowed my pace a bit. I'd rather think about trucks and the big guy behind this wheeler than death, so I hung in there with the eighteen-wheeler, going up the grade, side by side. I was having fun. I liked Jack Driven—imagined his looks—dark skin, long face, husky voice, heavyset build and huge arms, muscles stretching his grimy white T-shirt. I began to chant to myself, "Jack, Jack, he's my man; if he can't do it no one can. . . ."

At the hill's crest Jack pulled out ahead, moving forward down the grade's other side now. Two can play, I thought, as I switched to lane three from lane one (Jack in lane two) and passed Jack, going 82 mph and not even glancing over to see just what the semi trucker did look like.

"Jack, Jack, he's my man; if he can't do it . . ."

Everyone catches on to road talk fast if they care to listen (I'm not talking here CB lingo, I'm talking real road moves), so the truck's speed surged ahead too and again there we were side by side at 82 mph. It isn't easy to control a Jeep at that high speed and look over to see what's bearing down upon your side—but I did, figuring that people don't die on their way to writing wills. This guy, the trucker Jack Driven, was wonderful; better than most and I've played with many, though not most. Driven had straight black hair, his face was tanned and long rather than round like many truckers' and his T-shirt wasn't a T-shirt at all. Driven had a blue plaid long-sleeved shirt with the cuffs rolled up to his elbow. I could tell his arms were big by the size of the forearm. I loved Jack Driven's forearms: tight, muscular, protective though dangerous.

Looking at him, he must have been looking at me because from under that black hood came a loud deep resonant horn blast; Jack blew his horn, so to speak. It's not right for a lady to blow her horn back so I just smiled and pushed the speed up a couple of notches. Jack was cool, though; he hung back and simply waited for me to hang back too. I did—not wanting to lose him—and he dropped back even farther. I did again, finding myself more and more excited by his imagination on the road.

Our speed was almost legal when I realized that Jack Driven had his blinker flashing; he was getting off at the next exit, which would take him across the Richmond Bridge. I wasn't about to lose him and his way would get me to where I needed to go; it was longer, but certainly better.

Jack glided off the exit ramp first, well aware of my tailing him, and we headed on toward the bridge. I could see him glancing into his side-view mirror to locate my place and he seemed satisfied with it. As we approached the bridge the road widened to four lanes (two for each direction) and I took the cue to move alongside the groaning semi as we raced onto the bridge, which undulates its way across the S.F. Bay. Side by side, now not even looking at one another, we took over the bridge, no one else being able to pass. It was not particularly our purpose to hog the road; we were paying little attention to the desires of others out there this bright morning. As we reached the first peak Jack moved ahead, just a nose, and I took that to mean that I too should respond somehow—not necessarily as he did, but somehow. I chose to lie back and let him take the lead as we rolled down the rise-and-fall bridge-way. At the bottom of the dip Jack's brakes flashed twice, signifying that we were "on." So I took the statement and surged ahead now, passing him and moving directly before his bumper into his lane. I led the man now and he seemed to be enjoying it too. The two of us rode across the bridge like this—he on my tail—both of us moving at a moderately fast pace, but one that allowed for maneuverability. The bridge seemed to stretch out forever and ever before us as we played together over its course. To say that we were not making love would be absurd because both of us knew we were and neither seemed to be bored with the other. But as the bridge's length stretched now behind us and the end of its span was at our doors a smooth fatigue set in, as if we were growing spent. Spent, on the road, is not a bad feeling; it is, in fact, quite nice: peaceful and gentle with hums rather than roars. The bridge a part of our past now, the trucker and I felt close: we had gone through this together. And as we pulled up to the stoplight at the bridge's exit—he now alongside me, the light red—we stopped. I looked over at Jack Driven and he at me. The trucker winked and I smiled.

# Screaming Julians

## GRACE ZABRISKIE

"The smoke of myth rising from, let's face it, fires of reality raging *somewhere* would have it that men get off any old way, while only women care about context," he said, lying there, doodling around my left nipple with a warm finger. I think he was working up to something about how context was important to him too, but I was already going to give him that in spades. The cracked Mantovani on the stereo and the gardenia incense were his idea, not mine. Besides, I was trying to get off any old way, so I did a one-eighty and sucked his cock for him.

Biggish cock. Not the longest, just one of sweet God's thickest. Not short, now, not short by a good two inches; and where else does so little mean so much, unless you're talking microchips? I mean, take something just long enough to pee out of, add enough to walk through a locker room without a towel, put two inches on that and we're in the ball park. Not the longest, right? But already nice. A normal circumference on that and, well, fuck it, maybe you've never had a baby, or maybe he's got a great tongue and never had asthma. You wouldn't complain unless he beat you every time he'd stayed out all night.

And, like I say, this guy had girth going for him too. You really had to open wide to give him head, but on the other hand, you weren't so likely to get into trouble with your gag reflex. I thought of this woman I knew then, who used to come into the joint where I tended bar twice a week. We were both painters, so we usually talked about art—meaning other artists, materials, and reps—but lately all she wanted to talk

about was cocksucking, and her recent "feelings of fatigue."
She'd met some musician and had been "fellating" herself into
a slack-jawed wonder. Which was no wonder at all, as far as
I was concerned. She was into the "Cosmo method," which
apparently involved "keeping the lips stretched over the teeth
at all times," for Chrissake. It sounded tiring as hell to me.

Anyway, now I was sucking him, feeling pretty joyful and
creative about the transformation of his fragrant, stout, blue-
white shaft from matte to an opalescent satin sheen. I loved
the way both his cock and my mouth were staying hot, even
though I was coming up for air a lot and checking the finish.
I was going for high gloss.

Problem was, he was trying to pull me closer, wanting to
eat me in return. And I'm not much on tit for tat. Besides, he
didn't yet want to *enough*, it seemed to me.

"No," I said.

"Why not?"

"Not yet." I went down again and really gave it to him.
Some like it soft and some like it strong, but they all like it
hot and they all like it wet. I alternated between soft and
strong, concentrating on hot and wet. Silence for a while,
except for my favorite noises.

"When?" he quavered. You could tell he'd forgotten when
what but felt obligated to keep up his end.

I don't know why this is, but with one guy you don't think
twice about talking to his dick, and with another guy it doesn't
really appeal to you. I crawled up his belly, his chest, got tired
of sustained sinuous movement and discussed the situation with
his Adam's apple.

"When what?" I teased.

He sounded drugged: ". . . when . . . ?"

"Yeah, right. When what?"

He remembered. "Get it up here, I want to do it to you."

Uh-oh. "Do it?" I'm "doing it" to him, so he wants to "do it" to me? To my "it," in fact, which he probably thinks of as being "down there"? I'm losing heat fast. I decide to give him another chance.

"Why?" (This was the kind of question for which there were many possible adequate answers, almost any one of which would have reversed the dangerous flow of my blood from groin to brain.)

"Why *what*?" he chose, lurching into a sitting position. "Shit." (My front tooth had just put a dent in his collarbone.) "Toothy little twat, aren't you?"

And then, as I thrashed about in rage, trying to get up, "Why do I want to eat you? Compulsive, verbal little bitch that you are? Why do I want to put my face between your thighs and kiss you everyplace but your clit until you're ready to beg me to do that little thing? Or until you start thrusting toward me, or until you try to grab my ears and put me where you want me? Why do I want to do that?"

During this speech, this music to my ears, he was methodically laying me back down again, gently extricating my legs from under me and separating them, one on either side of him.

"That's what you want to know?" he continued, beginning to play with my pubic hair with both hands, running his fingers through it, fluffing it, acquainting himself with the terrain beneath it, finding the cleft but declining to open it, sure that he could convince it in time to open on its own.

I remembered a midnight telephone chat with my brother during which I was ruing the lack of a feminine equivalent to "getting a hard-on," and he cleverly came up with "wide-on." (I remembered that only because I was getting one at the moment, not because I normally associate sex with my brother.)

Anyway, "Someday I think I'd like you to meet my brother," is what I apparently said at this point.

"Yes, baby, yes," he murmured now, nuzzling me with his nose, catching the ends of my hair between his lips and tugging ever so gently. "And someday I'd like you to meet my sister. She's verbal, very verbal, you'd like her. And beautiful—the way you're beautiful, and I've never really fucked her yet either. Maybe she'd like to meet your brother."

He needed some kind of talking to here, but I wasn't clear on what needed straightening out first: his attitude toward his sister, his attitude toward me, his general sexism, his—his tongue was doing incredible things. Once, untrue to his stated plan, his tongue flicked my clit, but only once. A minor slip, really, and just enough to . . . Actually, I felt pretty much like just shutting up for a while.

"Maybe the four of us could go somewhere for a long weekend together." What? Oh, he was still razzing me with the sibling business. I was starting to have trouble connecting. And dimly aware that I'd lost control of the entire situation. *Finally!*

Now, at last his lips closed for one warm wet instant around my swollen clit. And . . . sipped.

"Would you like that . . ." He came up and, taking his hands away from around—all around—everywhere his mouth had been, he slid them up my body and, cupping the undersides of my breasts with his palms, he touched my erect nipples, holding them between thumb and fingers, then pinching them, gently, relieving them and exciting them further. I felt my womb contract.

". . . someday?" He stared straight into my eyes for a moment, as though expecting an answer. From me, a slain kangaroo. I watched his eyes move over my breasts, my ribs, my abdomen, as his hands went back to where they were needed, and his mouth, eventually, followed suit. But not before I had noticed his lips purse and his jaw move as he looked at me, open to him, and realized that the sight had replenished his mouth with fresh waters. And then his hands and face were in me and on me in ways I had only dreamed of. At times there seemed to be no separation between his mouth and my cunt; I couldn't tell which was which; our membranes were continuous. He loved my cunt; he gloried in it; he forgot all purpose there but his pleasure. Twice I started to come and he knew it; took his mouth away and pressed his hand there; spoke, to divert me; touched my foot. This was no mechanical friction making, trying to get it over with, no cautious, localized "licking" and trying to stay out of trouble with God knows what all might be down there. He was drinking me; I was being drunk from, being eaten of, truly.

I'd been annoyed that he wouldn't say it at first—say that he wanted to eat me. I'd decided that if naming it gave him no joy or excitement, then neither would doing it. My impulse had been to "teach" him the word. Jesus. Now he was teaching me what the fucking word *meant!* Hmmm . . . "fucking" . . . Wonder what his version of *that* is . . .

And then the terminal feelings started, much too strong to put them off. No time to find all the energy, to make sure it would all be released, so I wouldn't have been irrevocably triggered but left unspent, half drained; tricked, in a way, and ready to kill afterward.

As powerfully and rapidly as my orgasm was coming now, part of my brain was registering that he seemed to know what was happening to me, as it happened, and to respond to each stage. As my body went rigid, he became frenzied at first, then checked himself as he intuited that this would worry me, distract me. I think now that he asked me what I wanted, needed, and that neither question nor answer was verbalized, but I heard:

"Tell me . . . tell me, baby."

And I must have answered, begging him to suck, please, suck it out, suck my clit, suck it out... because that's what I needed, and that's what he did. He sucked my clit, sucked it somehow in time with the waves, and I came and came and came and came, on and on, with all the goodness there that had grown into force, and tension, energy, power unusable for anything now but to come and burst forth from my brain and my spine and my cunt, and he never stopped; he sucked it all out of that long, long duct, that channel from brain to cunt. And he knew what was coming and what he was getting, and it engorged him beyond all endurance. So gruffly and lovingly that tears stung my eyes, he told me to hold on... hold on... and just as the last wave I could possibly stand was taking me under, he entered me, unerringly, his arrow finding its wound already made and dying to be made more serious.

"Oh, my God," I breathed, as I felt him come in, hold... then stroke, and hold... stroke, and hold with such controlled and utter passion that I came yet again, and then again, as he held himself in me, still, like God with a shaft of radiant energy creating some universe.

Sex like this takes me beyond love: I become religious.

It was much too soon to know if I loved him; I didn't even know if he liked my paintings yet, or what—if anything—he did for a living. (I prayed it wasn't this; few people with money liked my paintings, and I doubted that I could afford him.)

But I knew I adored him... and then, dear God, he came. And he screamed. Throughout his coming, he screamed. I came unglued. Shit! This wasn't going to be easy.

My only other lover who screamed when he came was Julian, and as far as I can tell now, I'd adored him for that alone.

He was beautiful—and English—and the worst lover I'd ever had. Julian never loved me, never made me come, never even tried. "I *can't* love you," he'd whined, having screamed himself out one night. "Can't you see I'm a complete emotional cripple?" I'd met him at a rock festival in Atlanta and followed him to New York and through three communes in the Bowery before he finally got rid of me, and I pined for a solid year afterward, dreaming of his fucking screaming spunk.

Well, now I was lost. We lay there as dead for a while, without even the energy to summon breath, trusting that our hearts were still beating. I remember being aware that my eyes were crossed and not having the will to focus them.

Then I tried to take a deep breath—too soon; some reflex made me belch. I started to laugh, moved slightly, and my cunt expelled the air it had gobbled, sounding exactly like a fart and shocking the hell out of me. Jesus, I was coming apart.

I looked at him with my probably still crossed eyes. He was laughing, mercifully ungrossed out, loving it. I attempted a smile.

"What have you reduced me to here?" I said. Or someone said. It didn't sound like my voice.

"I think you've just been born again," he said, leaning over and kissing my navel. "I'll get a towel. Don't get up, your ass'll fall off."

I watched him go to the bedroom door, watched it close behind him and the deep cleft of muscle he paraded on each buttock. My eyes drifted to the window, the grays and purples of late sunset. It's still day, I thought, still the same day. And then I heard the Mantovani record stuck on one particularly repugnant pseudocrescendo and realized that it had been doing that for some time.

What was going on? I might have fallen in love with him anyway, but this screaming business confused things. Why did it strike so deep a chord in me?

On the other hand, I reasoned, why did the struck chord

strike me as being so weird? This was no worse than a man's going nuts for nurses, or black panties, or . . . well, all that really weird shit some men go for. Hmmm. No comfort for me in this line of thought.

Maybe what I'd loved about Julian was something else, like . . . well, something else. And now I was needlessly associating the way he *came*, for Chrissake, with hopeless adoration—with disaster.

Somehow it seemed very important to go back over everything that had just happened. How exactly had I felt before he screamed? Had I loved him then? With his lousy taste in music and his dopey dumbass gardenia incense? Because I loved him now, goddammit, and if the screaming had done it, then I wanted out immediately. Fast. Before it was too late.

He appeared with the towel slung over his dick, which was, for this trick, erect. Again. Or still. Who cared? He was an unbearable show-off. A mere athlete. (I'd just managed to get my eyes uncrossed.)

I stared at him unpleasantly, trying to make the towel fall down. It held there a moment, then fell rather abruptly. Good. I won that one. We both stared at the towel on the floor.

"Don't you want the towel, Julie?"

Great! *Perfect* timing! He hadn't used my name before. And, fortunately, he still hadn't. My name isn't Julie.

"Julie, huh? Is that your sister's name? Julie?"

He look surprised. "Yeah, it is. As a matter of fact. How'd you know that?"

"I don't know," I said airily, "just lucky I guess. Actually, I'm psychic. Notice how I made your towel fall down?"

"Yeah, I noticed. Bet you can't do that twice," he leered, moving toward me, pink towel preceding on its ever-rising flagpole. I snatched the towel, and, with mixed emotions over having so soon to leave its country forever, began mopping up with it. From my kneeling position on the bed I jerked my head at the stereo.

"Look, could you do something about that record?"

He turned off the stereo.

"Thank God. And could you open a window? This gardenia shit is driving me up the wall."

"Really?" he said, struggling with the window. "Harry told me at the party that you loved it."

"*Gardenias?*" I said, incredulously, but I was finding his manner most interesting. He was refusing to rise to my bait, yet I knew he wasn't afraid of a fight.

"Yeah. Well, he said you told him you used to babysit for some people who had Mantovani records, and so that music reminded you of necking over there with your first boyfriend late at night after you'd put the baby to sleep. And I don't know ... something about the smell of gardenias."

"Harry told you that?"

"Yeah, I saw you at the party and I wanted to meet you. Harry said no I didn't ... because your name was Julie. See, he had a thing for my sister in college, and she dumped all over him. I was going with a girl named Julie too, and when she dropped me for her German prof, Harry and I used to get drunk together a lot."

Somehow he was telling me that whatever had happened to us years ago was powerless to hurt us now. His past loves might be of interest to me, but not threatening. It occurred to me that—if I hadn't been about to end this relationship in a few minutes—I could probably in time have learned to tell him my stories with their true original flavors. *That* would have been a new experience. He was suggesting an area of mutual trust that intrigued me ... but I decided to concentrate on trying to piece this mess together. He was sitting next to me on the bed, sort of helping me with the towel.

"Yeah?" I said. "And . . . ?"

"Okay, so I'd been looking at you for about an hour, and you'd looked at me a couple of times too, right?" (Nobody needed this much help with a towel!)

"Right," I said, moving his hand away.

"Right, so I pointed this out to him. A name was a name, I said. Big deal. I liked you, I could tell you liked me too, so introduce us, Harry."

"I see," I said. "And that's when he said that he happened to know you could knock me off my pumps with Mantovani, so if I ever came here, you should have some waiting? So when you were coming out of the morning showing of that vile film—which you didn't even *warn* me about as I was going in for the matinee, by the way—and invited me to come over here after the show for a glass of wine . . ."

"I *liked* that movie," he interrupted languidly from the crook of my arm, which he'd grabbed and begun kissing and then licking a little. "Sorry there wasn't any wine."

"Oh, that's okay," I said, retrieving my arm, which was beginning to zap megavolts to my cunt. "You were busy running around to every used record store in town trying to find these clinkers. Weren't you?"

"Well, no, actually I didn't have to—"

"Let me tell you something, Ben. Your name *is* Ben?"

"Yeah, that's what Harry calls me—"

"Good. Funnily enough, though, no one calls me Julie."

"What do you mean?"

"I mean my name's Barbara. Listen, the first time I met Harry, he invited me to come over to his place and listen to his goddam Mantovani records. I said no way, not even for laughs. It *was* a high school story, but it's kind of bass-ackwards from what he told you." I wrenched whatever he'd got hold of next away

from him and started pacing. "Gardenias he threw in for free.
So. Your old buddy set you up for a fall, and you got laid
anyway. And all it cost you was—" I rifled through the stack.
"Jesus, Ben, how much *did* seventeen Mantovani records cost
you?"

"Come here," he said, "and I'll tell you."

"Oh no. I'll tell you. You didn't have to buy them; you
already had them. I get it. Harry turned you on to Mantovani,
you turned Harry on to your sister, and two of them turned
you on to your substitute Julie, and then it all fell apart and
nobody's been the same ever since. Ben and Julie and Mantovani and Harry and Julie... *Où sont les neiges d'antan*, right,
Ben?"

"Julian."

"*What?*"

"What's the matter?"

"What are you— Are you are you telling me *your name's*
*JULIAN?*"

"Don't shriek, Julie—"

"MY NAME IS BARBARA! MY NAME IS NOT—"

"I mean Barbara. Calm down; what's the matter? Look; Harry
calls me Ben. For Benjamin. My name is Julian Benjamin, okay?
... Where are you going?"

I was overreacting. And where I was going was to do more
of that in private. But now he'd caught up with me, holding
me close from behind, mumbling some nonsense about how I
didn't have any clothes on. I knew that! His hands were on
my breasts and I could feel his big hard cock in the soft small
of my back. And suddenly I wanted it in me more than I wanted
to get away. (I could always get away later, I reasoned.) So I
turned around and put my arms around his neck, and then his
mouth was on mine, and he was helping me climb him, pulling
one leg up around him; but not then, not yet. First the other

leg too, his hands holding me out from him then pulling me in, softly imbedding himself within me, deeper and deeper, then holding still till his sweet scream came, tearing out of him, into me, and I came then, before he'd finished . . . and *that's* never happened, before or since.

Three days later we were still there. At Harry's. (It was Harry's place, of course, and of course they were Harry's records. Ben was staying there, waiting for the loft to be rewired over his art gallery.)

I uncrossed my eyes, took a mercifully uneventful deep breath and asked if I could call him Ben.

"Why? Hey, what's the deal with my name?"

"It would just be better—for both of us—if I didn't have to call you Julian, okay?"

"Well, dammit, it's my *name*, and it— Oh, I get it."

"You do?"

"Well, you freaked out because I thought your name was Julie, or because I once had a girlfriend named Julie, or because you thought I wanted you to be my sister, or I don't know what the fuck, but anyway, I get it. Some guy's name was Julian, right? That asshole you used to babysit for?"

"Uh-uh."

"Oh, Jesus . . . your *brother's* name is Julian?"

I shook my head.

"Tell me."

I didn't like this.

"*Tell* me, goddammit. I want to know!"

I remembered our so far somewhat unilateral area of mutual trust, but had an uneasy feeling that this story should remain an exception. I wavered . . . and went for it.

"Look, Ben, you know how you scream sometimes, well—"

"What?" he interrupted, looking genuinely puzzled.

"When we make love, baby, and you—you know, scream?"

"I scream when we make love?"

"Well, when you come you do, sort of, you know."

"Are you telling me that I scream when I come? Like"—and he screamed then, a weak little falsetto scream, nothing like the real thing. And he was laughing. He honestly had no idea what the real thing was. He'd never heard it. What if telling him made him hear it? What if it made him stop? I had to get out of this. He'd stopped laughing.

"But what does screaming have to do with Julian? Come on, whatever it is, you're going to get over it, so what is it? Who was this Julian, and"—laughing again—"what's this about screaming?"

How the *hell* was I going to get out of this? Screaming. Julian. Two of them. Screaming Julians... SCREAMING JULIANS! TWO Screaming Julians! Well, I'm a bartender—and a bartender's daughter, as a matter of fact—and that sounds like a drink order to me.

So, I told him the truth: about how there was, uh, there was this waiter, this, uh, weird screaming faggot waiter named Julian who worked at my father's bar in New Orleans (I'd already told him about my father's bar), and I, uh, *hated* him, but my father thought Julian was JUST GREAT. Named a drink after him. Which became fairly well known, and then right after that my father died. Pretty traumatic stuff. And so the name, you know, freaked me out, and I always dreamed of him screaming.

"Who?"

"My father... And, uh, Julian."

"Oh."

And then the weirdness with the name Julie. Just too much. He bought it. For a minute.

"Yeah, but why does all that make you think you hear *me*

scream, Barbara? Well, I mean, I don't know what I do. Do I really scream?"

"*No*, no, you don't scream, not . . . *scream* . . . it's just that the first time we made love, you made some kind of noise . . . you did, really, and I fell in love with you then, I mean that day, and I guess in my subconscious mind, when you said your name was Julian . . . it got all mixed up . . . in my subconscious mind."

He was nodding now: he understood. Even I understood. I was even ready to forgive that fucking waiter.

"Can you make one?"

"What?"

"A Screaming Julian. Harry's got some of everything in the kitchen; why don't you go and make us a couple of Screaming Julians, and then we'll drink them, and then I'll fuck your eyes out."

"Ben, I don't know if I can—"

"Just go on in there and poke around. It'll come back to you; hell, they were famous, right? Somebody must have said what was in them."

I did it. I whipped them up. They were great. Ben says as long as I fuck him four times a day and feed him Screaming Julians I can call him anything I want to. I call him Ben. (Harry now calls him Julian, but we don't see Harry much. Except at gallery openings, when we serve Screaming Julians. Harry calls them Flaming Fucking Julies, but that's Harry.) And Ben says he'd still love my paintings, even if they didn't sell so well— in his gallery. But, hell, after a few months with Ben, I was *painting* well. So I guess you could say he screams for a living. But he still doesn't know it. Isn't that funny? Men are like pornography, in a way. They're amusing, but you still get off on them.

# THE PHYSICAL

## The Work to Know What Life Is

### DEENA METZGER

At night, when you were in my body,
when you were the tree giving breath to the night,
I took it in. We lay there,
your mouth open against mine
with the breath going back and forth.
I said, "This is the Amazon.
I want to grow dark as a jungle with you,
to feed all the myriad birds,
to give off air to breathe."
We lay together, dark woods feeding the universe,
you breathing into me,
I, taking your breath, holding it in my body, saying,
"Life, Life, Life."

I wanted to be a plant form.
I wanted to laugh under you like grass,
to bend and ripple,
to be the crisp smell,
to be so common about you,
to be everywhere about you,
to house the small and be there under your body
when you rolled there where I was.

*   *   *

I wanted to be the animal form,
I wanted to howl,
to speak the moon language,
to rut with you as the August moon tipped toward roundness
and the blood poured out of my body.
I held your penis that had plunged into me
and afterwards, my hands were red with my own blood,
I wanted to paint our faces,
to darken our mouths
to make the mark of blood across our bodies
to write, "Life, Life, Life,"
in the goat smell of your hands.
You carried it all day on your fingers
as I carried your pulse in my swollen cunt,
the beat repeating itself like a heart.
My body had shaped itself to yours,
was opening and closing.

I wanted to be the forms of light,
to be the wind, the vision,
to burn you like a star,
to wrap you in storm,
to make the tree yield.
I wanted to drown in your white water
and where your fingers probed,
I wanted to hear each pore cry out,
"Open, Open. Break open!
Let nothing be hidden or closed."

I wanted to be all the violences of opening,
all earthquake and avalanche,

and the quiet,
all the dawns and dusks,
all the deep blues of my body,
the closing and opening of light.
I wanted to be the breath from the lungs of the universe
and to open your mouth with a tongue of rain,
to touch all the corners and joinings
and when you entered me,
when I heard you cry, "Love me, love me,
love me with your mouth,"
I wanted to enter you with everything wet and fiery,
to enter you with breath
until you also called out
and called out and called out,
"Life, Life, Life."

# The Drainage Ditch

## GISELLE COMMONS*

It's late spring and we are helping friends by pickaxing a drainage ditch behind one of their buildings. Since I have never
used a pickax before I spend some time locating its balance,
my center. We alternate axing and hauling away the water-
soaked muck. The soil is red clay, somewhat rubbery, sticks
to our skin and clothes in bright splashes.

We touch each other intimately as we pass in the narrow
gully between bank and building. During one break we start
to neck. She goes to pee into the can on the porch, returns,
gloves in pockets, fastening her pants. Lasciviously I rub my
heavily clothed labia against her bent and braced thigh, caress
taut nipples, pushing through her shirt. Shifting, she opens
my pants, slides her hand inside and down, spreading my legs
wider. My boots slip in the mud. She tightens her grip around
my waist until I regain my balance. I prop one boot against
the wall and press against her, hungry.

She slips inside me, starts to fuck me quick and hard, her
knuckles rubbing firmly on my glans. I wiggle my torso back
and forth, up and down, more, more. She whispers encouragement: "Yes, yes, love, let it come." I feel like I'm pulling
everything into my pelvis: her fingers, my labia and my asshole. I hold my breath for as long as I can, gulp air and hold
my breath again, think I can't maintain this tension much

*Giselle Commons is the pseudonym used by the author for her erotic writing.

186

longer. All of my being is wound into one tight ball, somewhere in my middle.

With that wonderfully intuitive awareness she has about me she knows where to touch and how to move, knows I'm going to peak soon, gazes at me soft and open, rubs my clitoris with her thumb. I close my eyes again and wait in that quiet, hollow-feeling place until I see the flames licking out behind closed lids, feel my shoulders hunch and then convulse. Shuddering, I come and come.

Slowly I return, clinging to her, breathing in heavy short gasps. The odors of sweat and love mingle with smells of damp wood and sun-warmed grass. I kiss and lick her salty neck, push her gently against the building, work my boots more firmly into the clay. We kiss for a long time before I go in search of her wetness. She sighs as I enter her, rest there for a while then bring the moisture out and up around her pearl. Moaning, she turns her head from side to side, draws me on with the darting pelvic thrusts which I find so exciting. I flatten my fingers, move them between her inner lips, rub my face and lips against her cheek.

Her knees begin to wobble. I grasp her leg with mine, push her more firmly against the building with my weight. She presses her mons hard against my fingers till I reach inside with short deep thrusts. Oh how wet she is, I sing inside, I tell her she is very wet. She rocks upon my fingers, then brings my hand out again. I return to her hooded lady, rub the head and shaft with slippery silken fingers, separate the hairs.

Her head is thrown back, neck arched forward, shoulders shaking. Little quakes run up and down her body, she starts to vibrate all over. I am full of loving her, wanting her joy. She quivers, then seems to shatter around my cupped and writhing fingers, vagina opening to me, clenching around my knuckles in thigh-squeezing bursts.

In her cabin that evening we talk about our afternoon loving, linger over favorite moments, warm and close. Turned on again, I tense my heavy limbs and clasp her leg between my own. We rub and talk and tease until we both come again, fingers and toes curled tight. We laugh and hug, amazed at this river of passion that runs beneath us, rising to our surface and taking us, sometimes abruptly, giving little warning of the depth and power that will surge and crest, subside and leave us shaken and spent.

# THE CONTEXT

## *Tropical Places*

### UNSIGNED

The years speed by, but three lovers always will be remembered with a Cheshire grin. Alone in bed with closed eyes, my thoughts float backward to my life as a journalist and the men of tropical places.

FRANZ OF LAMU. A journalist traveling by dusty bus up the Kenyan coast—Mombasa to Mokowa. Two months writing about the Jews of Ethiopia and Israeli aid projects in Kenya. An ancient wooden boat rows me to Lamu, the site of an Israeli-run handicraft center. On this feudal African tropical isle, hidden in the Indian Ocean, women are covered in flowing black "buibui," while their protective Moslem men, also dressed in black, leer at the few foreign women. I sat on the veranda of the small hotel sipping the morning's mango juice. Five pink-skinned strangers beckoned from the beach below. I joined them and we became an instant brotherhood in the Swahili sea. No clocks, no telephones, no schedules; we agreed to a boat picnic outing to a nearby island.

Six strangers armed with oars, suntan oil, mangoes, pineapples and Nikons off to conquer an island for an afternoon. Giggling strangers in another man's land smiled a *"Jumbo, habai gani!"* greeting.

We swapped travelers' tales. André's told in sexy French-accented English; Kayoko's in delicate embarrassed Jinglish; Luigi's with animated Italian gestures; Anne's in loud Australian ebullience; me, the expatriate American, passport bulging with multicolored visas; and finally, the quiet man with the sensitive emerald eyes. I wanted to know this man. His strong, intelligent face was full of expression and character, masking no emotion.

But when I heard his deep voice utter sounds of guttural German, my interested smile froze. I smelled the ovens of Treblinka, I heard the black boots marching, I saw the shops with "Jüden" smeared on the doors. I felt rage building. I would not forget and I could not forgive. His people were responsible. Why did he have to mar the comradery of our tropical sea odyssey? I ignored him. I grabbed two oars and rowed furiously. I listened to the others laugh as Lamu became a distant hump hidden in the waves.

We neared Pate Island, rowing past a miniature fishing village to a deserted cove. Lying on the powdered sugar sand, browning our bodies, we ate, leaving lips sticky with pineapple. Massaging our bodies with warm coconut oil, we peeled off bikinis, trunks, our outer skins. They were no longer necessary. We were no longer strangers.

We waded into the cool azure liquid, a relief from the brutal tropical sun. Splashing, we played our bodies deeper into the water. The Australian suggested we race to a nearby atoll.

Five... four... three... two... one! The group broke into six lone swimmers. We were competitors now, intent on passing each other. With a burst of strength, I plunged ahead, right behind the German. He and I sleekly knifed through the water. We moved farther ahead of the others, our strokes stronger and faster.

Then Luigi announced, "Enough!" and leisurely floated back to shore. I swam intensely and with a burst of energy neared the German's kicking legs. No German was going to outdistance me, a California surfer. I twisted my head back; all the others were heading back to the beach.

The German and I were alone in the ocean. We surged on. I turned off my mind, letting the power of my legs and arms take over. I squinted ahead. The atoll was no closer, but our island of friends was receding far behind. My body was becoming heavier and heavier, inching more slowly through the now unfriendly thick water. I was getting listless, but nowhere to rest. The German was far ahead, swimming in easy, even strokes. I felt the vast ocean sucking me down. I had to move or I would be swallowed up. I yelled to him. "Franz!" Finally, I'd uttered his name. My screams tore through the silence.

He heard. Turning, he lapped toward me. He stroked my arm reassuringly. "It's okay. I'm with you now. Nothing to fear." I needed him. I was afraid, exhausted, my tears one with the water. He held my waist and relaxed me into a float. He coaxed my panic away and I felt the strength slowly returning to my hands, my arms and my sluggish legs. I languidly moved forward, Franz by my side. We inched ahead and when the water became translucent, my spirits soared. I spotted colored fish darting in and out of the coral castles. The atoll was getting closer.

When my feet felt the sandy bottom, tears of repressed fear were released again. I could barely walk. But the German's grin wiped away my painful drama. We faced each other, our bodies naked, no longer swathed in blue water. He tenderly brushed strands of wet blonde hair from my face. "What a delicious way to meet," said his eyes. I felt shyly naked with this man with the strange name. We were very much alone.

"We swam at least six kilometers and now we're stranded."
I didn't answer. Sensing my discomfort, he offered his bandanna, which he'd kept tied around his neck. I didn't know
what to do with this ludicrous piece of cloth with its red
cowboy design. I giggled at the absurdity. We were on an
unnamed atoll, off the island of Lamu, off the coast of Kenya,
somewhere in the Indian Ocean, far from anywhere, and a
German was offering me a red bandanna to cover my naked-
ness.

We could do nothing. We couldn't explore the atoll. Probably uninhabited, but if not, we would find Moslems—and
we two naked infidels. I thought of the others, picnicking
without us. Their sun-glazed eyes couldn't see us. We were
forgotten.

I studied him. Again he was a Nazi, a Jew-killer, and I, a
naked Jew. We sat under a palm and he began to talk. But as
I listened, this German became an intriguing man, a man I
wanted to know. He ceased to be Nazi and I forgot our na-
kedness. An architect, he'd been working in Zambia for four
years, helping house the homeless. A Berliner, he was also a
man of the world, a German Zorba with brains and guts.

I was drawn to him and he sensed it. Our rush of words
stopped. He moved closer. Drinking in the message in his
eyes, I inched back, afraid, yet wanting.

"Franz, I must know. Your father. What is he doing now?
He was a Nazi during the war, wasn't he?"

"My father was a doctor, a surgeon."

Dachau? Auschwitz? Another Dr. Mengele, another angel
of death experimenting on my relatives in the death camps?

"He was taken prisoner during the war. The Nazis called
him a Communist and shot him in the head."

I moved closer, pained and angry at myself for my ugly

thoughts. My fingers touched his face in apology. We fell silent, watching a gull loop and turn in the African sky. All other words forgotten, we now shared ours.

I felt comfortable. I let myself be in this place in this time with this man. I returned his inviting gaze. As our lips met, Franz whispered, "We're going to discover much more than this island now."

Our desire was magnetic as he drew my body close. Gently, he covered my neck with kisses. Our mouths met in longer and stronger kisses. An urgency was building as our bodies merged and I relaxed in his embrace. His tongue gently teased my right nipple. As he caressed me, I loosened to him, enveloped in the feeling, touching spell. I wanted this man.

I studied his dark hair spread across his flat, muscular stomach. My hand cautiously explored his penis, a throbbing testament to our mutual desire.

His strong hands worked their way down my thigh. I felt his fingertips gently touching and circling the wet lips of my vagina, making me shiver with each wondrous sensation. We had to have each other—now.

I closed my eyes and moaned as I felt him enter me. He was thick and strong and deep inside me. We communicated beyond words, our bodies speaking in long, slow movements in perfect unison. It was as though we'd always been lovers. As my body kept rushing in a sexual flood tide, he increased his thrusts.

I was about to explode. I was near the edge. Our hips pushed to the limits of passion. I shivered in delight as he slid his hand between our bodies, caressing my clitoris with stronger, faster strokes. We were both breathing heavily, both holding off the ultimate. Then I couldn't hold any longer. I burst into another plane of fiery sensation. Plunging into the swirling oblivion of orgasm, my fierce jerks welcomed his explosion.

Ecstatic, we squeezed each other in joyful mutual climax. I clung to him, my legs wrapped around him.

The African sun blazed down on us. We were one.

MICHAEL OF MOEN. A journalist traveling by Air Micronesia, the small plane patiently circling the tiny airport in its weekly ritual. The Moen islanders chased their pigs and sheep from the coral runway and we landed. Armed with a tape recorder, I was to get the story of twelve Tawabati islanders rescued after sixty-two days lost at sea. Their boat's motor dead, they had drifted 1,500 miles without food or water. Twenty-one had died before the survivors were plucked from the sea near Moen Island.

I checked into my hotel, a thatched hut, the only hotel on Moen. For a jungle lover, this five-mile island was tropical perfection, an untouched, unknown jade gem in the South Pacific. The largest of the Truk Island chain, it had no roads, telephones or electricity. I vowed to finish the assignment quickly and explore this paradise.

I trekked to the "hospital." Built by American aid, the three-story structure had no doctors, no medicine, no sheets, no soap—just a few ill-trained male nurses. The survivors greeted me with frightened eyes, silently staring from shrunken bodies. The malnourished children, their stomachs distended, lay on filthy cots next to gnarled fishermen. They had survived the angry sea for sixty-two days, but could they survive this moldy hospital? They spoke Gilbertese and these islanders, only Trukese.

I couldn't bear it. I walked down the hill to the general store and returned with bananas, oranges, soap and combs. I made the orderlies remove the Spam and Fanta. This was no feast for people who somehow survived on rainwater collected in coconut shells and sea turtles and fish caught with a string and pocket knife. It was a cruel joke, this modern hospital without medicine. They could have gotten better care from their village faith healer.

I stayed five days. Without even a first-aid course, I tried nursing them. We communicated by gestures and pictures. They didn't know where they were, only that they were far from their atoll in the Tawabati Islands.

On the fifth day I met him. I was walking toward the hospital and he was leaving it. He stoped his motorbike and watched me approach. This dark, burly, bearded man was Michael, an American doctor flown in from Guam to give help to the survivors. He was familiar with Moen, he visited it routinely as he island-hopped with his black medical bag around Micronesia.

"I've heard about you, journalism's Florence Nightingale," he said as he restarted the motor. "Jump on, I'm kidnapping you. We're going diving."

We entered the clear peaceful waters of the enchanting Truk lagoon, relieved to escape the reality of the hospital. We donned masks and tanks and discovered another world beneath the surface. A World War II graveyard, the lagoon was littered with Japanese submarines, many of them never opened. The Japanese had developed the lagoon into a naval base. Encircled by a reef and strongly fortified, it had been bombed by the Americans. The subs were now a silent testament to the raging raids and watery deaths.

Michael and I climbed onto our boat. Pulling off our masks, we realized we were still strangers. Diving partners who'd barely spoken, we were the only Americans on this tiny island. I was glad to share this tropical Garden of Eden with him. I liked his friendly, open face, his hearty laugh and his smiling blue eyes.

Michael handed me a flask of brandy. "Enjoy this because there's no booze here. The Moen men were the most violent drunks in the Pacific. Their women decided to bring prohibition to the tropics. They went to the polls one Sunday morning while their men were too hung over to vote. Democracy in action—the women won 100 percent. Booze is banned on Moen, so let's drink this precious liquid."

We shared a knowing smile. We both knew we were becoming more than friends. "So what do they do here?" I asked. "I've never seen anyone work. Certainly not in the hospital."

He fixed his gaze on me. "They make love. And when they're spent, they sit on the beach watching the waves and the sunset. They indulge in the only local produce—grass. They get stoned, they make love and they get stoned again."

He anchored the boat and snorkled around the magnificent orange coral reefs, trailing purple and green shimmering fish. I followed Michael to shore and the boat shed. "I have a surprise for you," he announced as he pulled out a long, delicate stick. "It's a love stick. Each Moen man carves his own, which he carries as his calling card."

"What's a love stick used for?" I asked, fondling it, half amused, half intrigued.

Michael moved closer, hesitated and then drew me close. Between kisses he explained, "When a man wants a woman, he waits until night and goes to her hut. Quietly, without awakening the other family members, he steals to the spot outside the wall where she's sleeping. He pushes the stick through the bamboo slats and waits for her response. She touches the stick, reading his Braille signature with her fingers. If it has the distinctive carvings of a man she desires, she draws the stick in through the bamboo and sneaks out of the hut. They find a hideaway and each other. If she doesn't want him, she pushes the stick out of the hut and he leaves, stick in hand."

Michael drew me to him as he outlined my lips with his tongue. I felt a rush of delicious anticipation. We walked the beach, talking, touching, knowing that soon we would have each other. But it was late and he was needed at the hospital. He roared off on his bike.

He didn't return. I wandered on the beach alone that evening. We'd shared a beautiful afternoon with a wonderful beginning and middle. But the end remained unwritten. Maybe I'd misjudged his interest. I felt empty, rejected.

The next morning I returned to the hospital, to the survivors, I told myself, but I knew I was there to find Michael. A nurse told me the doctor had left suddenly last night by motor launch to another island, where two men had been hurt in a fishing accident. I felt relieved. He hadn't left me, but I couldn't wait for his return. I'd finished writing my story and the weekly Air Micronesia flight was due that afternoon.

I thought of Michael and what might have been as I took one last walk around the island. I explored the abandoned Japanese bunkers and munitions dumps. The island's scars were everywhere: the War in the Pacific had left lonely skeletons, spent bullets and silent subs.

As I stood in the airport shack, I watched my plane circle for a landing. I should have left Michael a letter, I wanted him desperately now that I knew I could never have him. I watched the plane dip, lift up and then circle again. The pigs and goats wouldn't leave the runway. The impatient pilot had other passengers waiting in Panape and Palau. With a jerk, he took the plane up, leaving me staring at the sky. He'd given me another week on Moen. I was overjoyed, thinking of my reunion with Michael.

That evening, I leaped onto my bed, anxious to end the day with a deep sleep. But I sensed something. I felt a presence in the room but I couldn't see anything in the dark. Breathing quick, frightened breaths, I waited silently. Something was sliding through the wall. A viper? God, what should I do? I felt very alone, as I visualized the hidden serpent's fangs. I heard a muffled sound. I sat up. Something brushed my cheek. A thin piece of wood was coming through the bamboo wall. I felt the carvings on it and understood. A love stick! A muffled sound outside became a loud laugh. I pulled the stick into the hut as my heart beat rapidly in anticipation.

As the door opened, I suddenly froze. Why did I stupidly assume it was Michael? He'd left without a goodbye and didn't promise a return. What if it were some squat, stoned islander? All the Moen men knew where the American woman's hut was.

Nervously I demanded, "Who's there?"

"Can't you read the stick? It's me. I just sailed back. There was a terrible accident on a tuna boat." The outline of his enormous six-foot-three frame filled the doorway. As I leaped up to embrace him, he playfully pushed me back onto my bed. Pulling off my T-shirt, he kissed me passionately. He began working his tongue down my neck to my nipples, his wet slurping sounds amplified in the tropical stillness. His tongue moved expertly, as if he'd always known my body.

I worked my fingers down his chest, half tickling a trail to his inner thighs and to his penis. I saw its gleaming head rising urgently. He buried his face in my breasts, and at the same time, his fingers made gently encircling strokes of my clitoris— slow, then faster and faster.

Michael suddenly stopped and sat up, poised above my

body. He looked wanton and delicious. I closed my eyes in anticipation as his penis traced a path down my stomach, nudging between my legs. Then with a swift, strong stroke, he entered me. Then again and again, deeper and harder. My body arched, releasing itself from my mind. Michael's tongue moved in and out of my mouth in perfect unison with his penis. I let out a silent scream as my body prepared to erupt.

Abruptly, he pulled away. Seconds seemed like minutes, my body waiting, aching for more. Then, when I could stand it no more, he thrust in with precision timing, again and again, and again. Teetering on the precipice of orgasm, we could do this forever. Once more, he paused and waited for my body to scream for more, yearning to have him back inside. At the exact second, he thrust in for our shivering, quivering joyous mutual climax. Michael knew me that night. Exhausted and spent, we clutched each other closely.

The love stick fell to the floor.

PAULO OF MANAUS. A journalist traveling the Amazon with time to kill. The photographer still hadn't arrived. For the last four days, he telephoned his arrival, but each Varig flight from Rio arrived without him. Like many Brazilians, his calendar had no place for American deadlines. But I had no choice. I needed him, so I waited. The editors of *Jornal do Brasil* promised they'd chosen a top photographer for this potentially dangerous undercover job. We were to infiltrate Projecto Jari, a secret country within a country, owned by America's richest man, the eccentric eighty-three-year-old Daniel Ludwig. The size of Holland, Jari was closed to outsiders, especially journalists. Poverty-stricken Brazilians were flown in, lured to Jari with promises of glorious wages. Then, trapped

without money, in a hidden jungle slum, they became virtual
prisoners. They cut trees for the mammoth paper factory that
was built on a boat in Japan and transported across the world
to this remote Amazon outpost. The Brazilian government was
covering something up, some of its highest officials were involved. The story was big and I had no photographer.

Impatient and frustrated, I couldn't face another evening
alone in my dingy, depressing Amazonas Hotel room. A woman
alone in this moldy river port a thousand miles up the river
stays locked inside at night if she's not a prostitute. But I didn't
care anymore, I wanted to see people.

I wandered to a nearby restaurant. I ordered a black bean
soup and pushed it aside. I wasn't hungry. I stared at my book,
but the words remained on the pages. I wanted to get out of
Manaus and do my story. That's when I noticed him. At the
next table, the man in the beige safari jacket was sketching
intently. I drank him in. Large brown eyes, shiny black hair,
pure elegance, not a local from this rough frontier town. A
young Omar Sharif. I concentrated on him, caught his attention, then hid my gaze in the book. I smiled inwardly at my
success as I felt him approaching.

"What are you reading?" he asked in his charming Portuguese
accent.

"*Xana*. It's about the destruction of the Amazon."

With suspicion, he asked, "Why are you so interested?"

Suddenly wary, I realized I didn't know who he was. In a
police state, one shouldn't reveal anything. I'd almost blown
my cover before I'd even gone undercover.

"I'm just a tourist from California. I like to read everything
I can about the Amazon."

His face relaxed into a smile. "And I like to draw everything
I can about the Amazon. My name's Paulo and I'm also visiting

here for a short time. Would you like this?" he asked, handing me a pen-and-ink profile of myself. With a few expert strokes, his drawing had captured my profile. "I'm going to explore Manaus tonight. Would you join me? Reality can be more fascinating than a book."

I didn't need to answer. He knew I wanted to be with him, he knew how to read faces. "Have you seen candomblé? It's Brazilian voodoo. The West African slaves brought their rites here. There's a very special candomblé house in a *bairro* up the river; I want to sketch the ceremony tonight."

As the artist and I went to the dock, I was now glad to be in this moldy port at the end of the world. Paulo hired an Indian to take us by motorboat up the river. We sailed past the lush vegetation panting with the eroticism of crimson passion flowers and fragrant white Amazon lilies.

Our boat silently glided past a baby jacare-assu alligator, his eyes gleaming from the depthless inky water. Sensing my fear, Paulo drew me close. The Amazon was mystery and danger. Both it and Paulo were more intriguing than dreams.

The boat approached a small cluster of buildings on poles perched along the riverbank. We got out and immediately the hypnotizing pounding of drums drew us to the candomblé house, an abandoned rubber warehouse. The moment we entered, we were in another reality. The small room was filled with the scent of tuberose, cedar and sweat. On the altar were sacred feathers, magical beads, bowls of cornmeal—offerings to the gods. Five caged howler monkeys were shrieking to the clapped rhythms of the possessed women.

At least thirty women, all in white, were writhing, screaming, chanting to Iemanja, goddess of rivers and water. Black women, mulattas, Indians—they were souls on fire. Paulo and I watched in silent fascination as they journeyed out of their bodies, falling on the plank floor in trance, incorporating the various *orixas*.

Now other women standing along the walls joined in the frenzied candomblé dances. As they quickened their pace, whirling, jumping, tapping secret reserves of energy, Paulo sketched. He motioned me close and took off his silver *figa* necklace, placing the good-luck amulet around my neck.

"Now you're ready to go outside," he said. "You're protected against the evil eye." We wandered hand in hand into the thickness of the jungle, its blackness alive with the sounds of the drums. The Amazon, source of half the world's oxygen; without this jungle, the planet earth would suffocate.

We entered a cacao orchard and spotted a white canvas hammock hidden between layers of vegetation. It was strung between two lofty trees, and about it golden cacao fruit shining out from the green-black leaves.

Feeling a bit of the candomblé trance myself, I eased into the hammock. It swung back and forth and then settled. Paulo gently nudged himself in beside me. All was quiet except for the nearby sucking sounds of the river and the pounding of the drums. Our embrace was broken by a tremendous fluttering as a flock of hundreds of small parakeets rose from the jungle and disappeared.

Paulo caressed my face and silently kissed me. We held each other, the heat of our bodies matching the heat of the evening, his smell the scent of the jungle. His tongue ran along the side of my neck, his teeth nipped my earlobe. He lifted off my blouse and edged his fingers gently under my lace bra.

The hammock began to move. And as our bodies came alive, the swaying intensified until we tumbled onto the moist ground, our bodies tangled in a soft bed of vegetation.

We were flesh to flesh, lost in each other. Our lovemaking

was gentle, yet fierce. Each of us spurred on by the intensity of the other. Our bodies locked together in perfect rhythm with the drums, becoming one as we moved in rolling waves.

Our breathing quickened and the groans became louder as our bodies twisted and turned in the cooling mud. Paulo moved faster and faster, stronger and stronger, thrusting deep inside me. "I'm coming, I'm coming," he screamed, shattering the jungle stillness. I couldn't hold off. I felt his explosion set off my orgasms in rapid staccato succession.

Exhausted, we lay spent, our bodies glistening with sweat and mud. "Let's stay together," he said, becoming the passionate Latin. "We have something special."

I wiggled from his embrace, knowing I must sober both of us. "I'm meeting a photographer from Rio and we're leaving tomorrow for Projecto Jari." I didn't want to say those words. I wanted our emotions to torpedo reality. I wanted to stay with this artist. I fell silent, waiting for him to wave a hand and bring the magic back.

Instead of becoming upset, Paulo howled, loud deep belly laughs. How could he laugh when I'd opened myself to him, wanted him. He found it funny. He didn't care.

"We're not going to be passing birds," he said, pulling me close. "We're staying together."

"But I'm leaving when the photographer arrives."

"I know," he chuckled. "I'm the photographer."

# The Bull Dancer

## DEENA METZGER

Now as you are poised over me, initiating a rocking movement, as your weight shifts forward from your heavy thighs, the tension palpable in the small of your back, and heat begins to seep up into the air, I remember the old woman standing erect, proud, even defiant in the middle of the room which was the dark chamber of Pasiphaë the queen of Knossos. We surrounded her and drummed and chanted as she spoke. Against her white hair, the blood rising in her face became the dark moon against the clouded sky. She placed her gnarled fingers, nails still rounded like Cretan arches, the small moons white at the apex, against her breasts and held them; her palms were brass breastplates covering the white cloth of her Romanian blouse. And I put my own hands on my own small breasts, covering them momentarily against the memory, as if I could be covered against this moment when you will descend upon me like a great white beast.

When she was just a child, a man had stopped her in the field. She said he walked straight toward her, his hands stretched out before him, like a blind man looking for a wall, and he clutched at her like one plucking apples, one in each hand, each stem left on the limb and the small-leafed declivity in the apple like the navel in my belly where the leaves of skin fold over each other. The little apples, plucked, twisted, bitten till she cried, then the man left easily as a great wind retreats over the mountain leaving the remains of broken trees, limbs scattered, leaves everywhere in the wake of the storm.

Escaping the old country, she took only the blouse, his handprints barely washed from the white batiste embroidered with small delicate cross-stitching. She continued to wear similar blouses, this one covered with flowers and animals in parade, as if, finally, innocence might protect her, her white hair as delicate again as the first corn silk of the young girl. She never married. She feared men, she said, as she feared unseasonable weather, typhoons, dust storms, orchards and worms. She kept the storm windows on her house winter and summer. Once I saw an orchard gone back to seed, apples across the ground brown and sweet and here and there young saplings sporing from a random seed. The trees were old and unpruned. The land had become virgin again, that is, seemed ancient again, looked wrinkled, all handprints removed. The soil had the sharp and acrid smell of humus like the wet moss between the secret crevices of rock. And I pursued the smell; I rubbed my nose in it, alone, unashamed of being the animal in the ecstasy of scent.

You lean over me and I can smell the urgency of your body, the temperature changing in your mouth, and once again I place my hands against my own small breasts hiding them from your shadow and then I push my fists up against your shoulders as if to keep an animal at bay: cock, drake, cob, gander, ram, boar, stag, hart, buck, stallion, ox, sire, bull.

The old woman turned in the circle as we drummed trying to keep a heart pulse going. Her past stretched out from her like a white sheet. Her vagina was pure as the head of a nun. It was covered in white silk and gauze.

In Crete, the moon queen ordered a chamber built in the form of a white cow and Daedalus, the greatest architect of them all, set the wood feet precisely in the wet grass, so that the garnet cow eyes faced the sun as it fell from the mouth of darkness and over the raised tail the tawny moon of autumn strove up into the anointed sky. The white heifer shimmered with longing in the moonlight. The moon queen crawled into this cow bed to wait for the bull god, while, by the hedge, Daedalus and Minos the king spied.

There is also an old woman in me as I lie in the bed enticing your great weight. There is someone wise enough to wait in me. There is someone who has learned the stories. Above me, the moon tosses in its sleep, turns her face against the cloud, sighs, breathes out the light.

The old woman stood, dreaming before us. She had spent her life wrapped in white satin, she wore embroidered cotton skirts, sat with her broad thighs crossed against the night. She stood in the middle of the room, immobile, her hands breast-plates upon her breasts, then swaying ever so slightly, as if conjuring a memory, and a beat, she began the drum, daring it to enter her.

Crouching above me you know the rhythm.

She dreamed aloud. "Outside on the wall which surrounds this palace of Knossos, where the stone bull horns reach up-ward to guide the planets, an old man has placed his wooden pipes in a careful bundle and selecting one plays to the tourists, making a high-pitched plaintive sound such as might call a lamb. Toot. Maaa. Toot. Maaa. We are together in the after-noon light. Above us the crescent moon rises upside down and I know that if it touches the stone horns of the bull, the universe will be reborn. I feel so much yearning in the air the ovarian horns in my belly sound their own brass notes. His coarse fingers, broadened by stirrups and leather, trill on the holes in the body of the flute. With the small knife at his side, he has stripped the wood, carved each hole, then shaped the pipe to the music he desires. Beneath him the roots of the olive tree grope about each other in the dark earth. I sit beside him on the wall in my embroidered skirt, opening my lap as if it were a bowl to catch the sun."

The smell of the old woman, ripe and sharp, swept toward me as if the pipe song propelled it, as if the man had drawn it up out of her and were blowing it out through his mouth, musk saturating the air. As she spoke, I could see these two old animals, the air full of the beckoning scent.

"He leans toward me, pungent with the breath of goat, and asks me to lie down on the soft knoll enclosed by trees. He says he has used that bed before. I tell him I need pillows and a feather quilt at my age, that lying against him will be like sliding down the twisted oak. His rough hands, I say, will catch on silk. He's so bony, where will I rest these breasts? But he extends his hands and offers me two apples, red as nipples. He is the bull god."

"Look," she dreamed, "the bull god is coming. Don't you see him coming, see him filled with years of longing?" Her face transformed till pity rested about her mouth. "He is coming to me gorged as the tipped moon before a rain, the brimming pomegranate erupting on the limb, its hard casing ruptured by the insistent translucent seeds."

In the dream, I saw her asleep in the field on a grassy hummock and the moon covered her with a blanket of light. You would not think she was an old woman; in the light she was the young queen, or the wooden cow, bristling and hungry. The old woman dreamed and I saw the dream before me as if I were also the old woman standing, asleep and transported. The white bull came with his hooves dancing to the tune of a little wooden pipe. Everything the bull god touched turned white. There were no longer handprints on her blouse. I saw the old woman awakening, the bull's testes in her hand; swollen with all the years of waiting, they were like sweet fruits and the skin was bursting with nectar. The old man with the pipes played for them as they hummed together. "Listen," the old woman whispered, "the bull song is entering my mouth. I have waited for these apples all my life."

You come down upon me as if you were an animal. On the phonograph, the drumbeats increase, the flute melds with the drum. I take the flute into my body, it quivers ever so slightly with your breath; you are the drum, the beat begins in your feet, you hold the rhythm, the peat moss rises about us; compressed into dark bricks it will burn. The flute is just a breath, it arcs delicately, swirls, twists and trembles, soars and falls, and I fall with it trembling under your dark and steady heat.

This is how a man becomes a bull. It begins at the feet. The heels turn hard and the toes cleave where the foot narrows. The blood quickens, heats, ignites. The hoof slides against my ankle, chafing, as the blood quickens through the narrowing hairy calf. Your skin becomes a tough and smooth hide, the muscles in your buttocks ripple about the rising tail. I feel your knees straighten and I must lift myself toward you, then turn under your gathering weight, taking it in the small of my back and turning back, arching higher to lie spreadeagled in the cavity of a white cow, my knees pressed up against her haunches, my spine agitating against her white leather belly, the muscles shimmy and thrust me upward, to circle your great neck. Your back is straight, then gibbous, and your chest bows and presses against my breasts. Out of such hide, a drum is made. Your heart heaves against me in its skin sling. A muzzle presses, nips at my neck; the teeth, square and heavy, grind against each other as a beast sucks my hair. I reach up to brace myself, arms barely able to grasp your rough mane. Your breath is full of grass. You have neither hands nor fingers. I reach up

and press forward, my head buried in the brush, the pillows
turn to hay, forelegs on my shoulders you press us deeper into
the sod. I am afraid to open, moo fearfully, then grunt as your
insistent flanks thrust forward, penetrate. A ramus, a living
staff, a dark persistent root inserts itself into my flesh. What
is sucked up from the earth through these fierce limbs and
lured from the sky through the arch tail? What emerges in the
twisted double braid as you lunge forward, surging with a
spinning double fire as if what runs through you must run
through me as well? After the animal shiver, my flanks shudder
under white hide. The hump on your back swells in the stab
of moon releasing all its rainwater. Inside my belly the red
seeds of the thrashing bull god churn.

In me, a moon beast—god, bull, man—paws restlessly at
his corral.

The ancients lied. The young boys and girls, bare-breasted
and girdled at the waist, did not somersault across the back
of bulls nor did they use the sword. *We* enact the first bull
dance. The old woman removes her breastplates, her white
blouse, binds her waist with a raw-silk sash cradling her apple
breasts in the gold winding cloth. Then she lies down. The
bull comes again and again. We drum and drum. The old man
blows his pipe, each finger careful to close the holes then open
them again. You lean over me in the bed snorting and pawing
at the wet sheets. I raise myself to you, cutting my hands on
the erect crescent horns. The great white animal bears down
upon me. This is the arena and the dance.

Take me to the fields, let me grasp the pommel, lift myself
upon your heaving back and ride.

# POWER

## A Few Words on Turning Thirty in Marin County, California

### CAROL CONN

I am a bit shaky as I park my car in front of the wrought-iron gate. My fingers tremble as I nervously reread the invitation to a "night of timeless fantasy." This evening with two male "geishas" comes as a special gift from my friend Sharon for my thirtieth birthday—something that could only happen in Marin County, California. Though I try to walk nonchalantly through the entrance, my pace is governed by a pounding heart which has somehow become lodged in my throat.

True to their word, my anonymous hosts have left a trail of candles to flicker the way through an elegant but overgrown English country garden. I stop to take in the mesmerizing scenery before me. Just beyond the yard is Mount Tamalpais's regal profile. Fog cascades down the mountain's sides, ablaze with fiery shades of pink, orange and purple in the remaining moments of yet another exquisite Marin sunset. Somehow it seems to be an appropriate omen for a thirtieth birthday and the evening that lies before me. Whatever happens, it will be no ordinary celebration.

Just beyond the rustic gate, the garden is an explosion of color with flowers blooming in every conceivable hue. Down at my feet, emerald moss, deepening to purple in the fading light, frames each crumbling brick in a path worn with age.

211

Magnolia and honeysuckle blossoms perfume the breeze.

The evening has the texture of an intricately woven silk carpet. It must also be a magic carpet, for each deep breath soothes anxieties and my mind easily drifts as though propelled by the soft gusts. The wind stirs my dress, the fabric caressing my thighs triggers an involuntary shiver. Smoldering sparks are reignited, once again shooting up and down my spine. The magic carpet carries me back to an earlier interlude. Barely an hour ago, I was a sexual surfer, endlessly cresting on a delightful wave of pleasure with the assistance of my lover's steamy lips and probing tongue. The momentum stirs my womb and a drop of remembered passion trickles downward.

The sudden movement of bats overhead brings me out of this sunset reverie and I continue walking to a cottage that is every bit as quaint and rustic as the surrounding garden. The doorbell's faint jingle is sufficient to reduce my newly acquired calm to the anxious uncertainty of a sacrificial virgin.

The front door opens onto a room ablaze with candles, rendering the two men clad in short kimonos into dark silhouettes.

"Hello, birthday girl," they chorus softly.

I enter, defensively modest under the intensity of their gaze. Then I recall my lover, Fausto, and his unspoken jealousy when he realized I had made other plans for this evening. Since our relationship is what it is—meaning true Marin style: no demands, no commitment—he had no right to question why I would not be with him on the night of my thirtieth birthday. But the smug gleam in his eye as he left my apartment let me know that he did have some inkling as to the evening's activities.

His message was abundantly clear: no matter what I do with another man tonight (not one, my darling, two), Fausto's sultry presence could not be entirely supplanted. His Latin jealousy stirs within me, eliciting some new-found strength from an undiscovered realm.

I raise my head and take charge of these two geishas with regal bearing. Tonight I am a divine goddess who will realize her powers as two priests worship me with all the ritual and fanfare of an ancient pagan religion.

My holy robes? Sheer black stockings with a black-and-red garter belt hugging my thighs. Black silk panties, now moist with anticipation, cling like a second skin under a loose-fitting thirties-style dress. It has a deep plunging neckline with slits up the front and sides. Sensuous black rayon material provides a dramatic background for the red lips embroidered all over it. The evening's magic seems to make the lips come alive, for they shimmer and dance invitingly in the candlelight. Appropriate vestments for these two mortals whose gaze has now softened into adulation as each lifts one of my hands to his lips.

I watch them kiss my fingers with studied eroticism and something dawns on me. My power depends on how much I can keep these men off balance; how well I can play different forces against one another. Unconsciously I have already made my first move by making love to another man.

I ease my hands out of theirs and walk over to the bar, where a bottle of champagne is resting in a bucket of ice. I pause, expecting them to anticipate my every whim and fulfill it. I have no intention of seating myself on a barstool. As if kicked into action, they both rush over and help me onto my "throne." Only then do I become aware of tedious sounds emanating from the stereo. The music is entirely inappropriate.

"Gentlemen, I am dressed for jazz. Give me Charlie Parker or Billie Holiday."

This sets off another frantic rush but produces none of Bird's albums. Fortunately Lady Day is in the house and my geishas can save face. Soon her sweet, sad crooning fills the room. My hosts breathe a sigh of relief as I relax and begin to enjoy a glass of champagne, some black gummy hash and the whole situation at hand.

It is now my turn to examine the geishas. Alexander is a tall, blond beach boy type about thirty. He is muscular but slim with tantalizing long legs. Jeremy is a fortyish, short dark artist with almost sinister looks. He has a slight paunch and coarse chest hair curling around the lapel of his kimono. They gaze back at me with an appreciation and lust that seems far more appropriate for a B movie than a birthday party. I laugh because I am stoned enough to believe their dialogue will be sufficiently corny to go right along with the script.

"Ah, lady," sighs Alexander, as if on cue. "You are truly beautiful. A fantasy fulfilled; an exquisite stranger has come for an evening of total pleasure. A gift from the gods."

Fool! I am a goddess. The champagne and hash, however, are taking me out of the temple to a less sanctified place. Billie Holiday is still singing the blues, making me feel like a tragic, erotic, gin-soaked mamma in a seedy thirties bar with two slaves to do my bidding. My geishas flow right along with the action. Presently Jeremy massages my neck and shoulders and his fingertips ever so lightly rub my nipples, which are rigid to the touch.

Alexander parts my legs, softly stroking each thigh with exquisitely sensitive lips. He probes my clitoris through the silk panties with his bewitching tongue. I float on that magic carpet, lulled higher and higher off the ground by the delicious sensation of Alexander's tongue.

I close my eyes and mentally I am once again sitting on my

living room sofa watching my lover Fausto as his hands grasp my thighs while he buries his face in my cunt. His caramel skin has a satin sheen, smelling faintly of eucalyptus trees and sweet sea air. He growls as I writhe with pleasure. My body is ablaze as I drift back and forth between Fausto and these two adoring strangers.

I am once again the goddess of this birthday temple. The goddess knows that the men who seem best able to love and appreciate women treasure bathing their faces in cunt juices. And these utterly devoted priests worship my pussy. They savor me as an exquisite taste experience, right up there with a vintage cognac or beluga caviar. The faintly musty perfume of my womb is a primal aphrodisiac, and eating me out draws them back into the Garden of Eden. Wanting to crawl back inside to this paradise, they can only enter a tongue, a finger or a cock, but at least that promises them a moment of retreat from the world.

These geishas' satisfaction and salvation comes only from my intense pleasure. And I don't give a damn how long it takes. If I withhold my orgasm from them, they will only try harder. I pull back and let the tension build. After all, these mere mortals are here to do my bidding. If one gets tired... well, there's always another.

Yes, Billie Holiday herself would have approved of such intense loving. So I try to prolong the moment and seize that silken thread of ecstasy, forever walking an erotic tightrope until I fall off into a deep orgasm. I am as silent as possible while arm, stomach, calf and thigh muscles twitch to different tempos until they finally pulsate in unison.

When the internal explosions finally subside, I gradually float back into the room and feel my body once again become solid. There I am, actually lying on a barstool with legs draped over Alexander's shoulders as he kneels before me. He gazes from between my legs with supreme satisfaction. He buries his face once more, comes up for air dripping wet and rests a well-shaven cheek against my thigh. Only now do I notice that Jeremy has been supporting my back and head as I lie in this horizontal position.

Billie Holiday is still serenading us, the dress has risen to my stomach, panties pulled down to stocking tops. Jeremy helps me to sit up as I nonchalantly straighten my clothing and hair. I drain the champagne glass and look at them without expression. Their desperate need to know I am pleased is so obvious. Let them wonder.

I pick up the pipe, smile sweetly and whisper, "More hash, please."

I barely suppress a laugh as they busy themselves with my request. It is all so absurd and wonderful. My women friends should have ringside seats for this performance. I want them to see Alexander run his skilled hands up and down my legs, nibbling delicately on each foot.

Jeremy tries to give wet, passionate kisses but I turn away. I sense the sting of rejection but the music, drugs and my emerging power preclude compassion. Besides, I find him overbearing and clumsy compared to Alexander's light touch. Jeremy must content himself with fondling my left hand.

The next glass of champagne is sipped in a bubble bath. Alexander carries me into a candlelit bathroom and tenderly takes off what little remains of my original costume. His hands and mouth are completely attuned to their task. Gently scrubbing my legs and feet, he covers each foot with kisses. Alexander seems perfectly content to play out my fantasy and I am totally content to let him.

He administers more hash and champagne amid a blur of

flickering candles against the bathroom tiles. When I emerge from that glorious bubble bath, he tenderly wraps me in big towels and then brings out a lilac silk kimono for me to wear. Apparently we are dressing down for dinner.

Alexander scoops me up in his arms and walks back into the living room. We snuggle together on a comfortable chaise longue. He continues his leg massage and I pray he will never stop. What a blessing: turned on, brought off and not required to give anything in return. Utterly selfish for an evening and no obligatory atonement. A Cheshire cat's grin spreads across my face as Jeremy brings food to the dining table across the room. It is rather an odd family meal we three sit down to. My geishas scarcely touch their plates and gaze at me with the same ardor I reserve for the chilled cucumber soup, lightly seasoned with fresh dill and mint. The clean crunch of cucumber mellowed with sweet yogurt, prepared by Jeremy, is seducing my taste buds. I see him sigh with relief and grow comfortable as I feed both him and Alexander artichoke leaves dripping with garlic butter. Alexander goes wild as I slowly pull a second leaf from his mouth; the sensuous scraping against his teeth, he says, recalls the sensation of losing himself between my legs shortly after I arrived.

The momentum builds as we ravage a leg of lamb glazed with a sweet, tart juniper berry sauce, roasted to perfection, tender and juicy. We tear the pink flesh with our hands in utter abandonment, rivaling the intensity of our encounter earlier in the evening. Alexander kisses away the meat juice trickling down my arm.

We regain some composure with the salad and sedately munch endive and Bibb lettuce. The understated dressing and crisp texture have a sobering effect, like swimming in a cool mountain stream. It not only cleanses our palates, the salad also clears our minds and bodies, making way for the upcoming event, which is my true incentive for consenting to this soiree.

A massage by two men. I have always wanted to feel four (or more) hands overwhelm my body with a soothing, healing touch. Alexander escorts me into a bedroom with so many candles glowing that in my present state the four walls look like a miniature Milky Way. Lilting Persian love songs cast an eerie mood, as if the ghosts of ancient lovers have come back to witness this act. Perhaps each tiny flame represents the soul of some great and passionate lover. Soon I am floating, levitated by four hands which skillfully assuage all tension. I am so moved by my geishas' tenderness and artful touch that it is hard to conceal my pleasure.

While Alexander continues the massage, Jeremy is now getting his long awaited chance to eat me. Despite his grasping personality, he knows how to explore the valleys and hills of my cunt with technical expertise. My body tenses up for another explosion but the goddess is determined to conceal it. Jeremy will never know. It is a totally contained energy when I do climax, like fireworks spreading sparks as silent as falling snow.

Now I am spent. Three intense sessions this evening plus a massage is enough to put me to sleep. I want to go home now but the hash, wine and champagne have precluded driving. How could I possibly stand up, get dressed and bid a swift adieu to my hosts? Too much trouble so my mind drifts on, savoring the massage. I am awake enough, however, to feel Alexander's cock enter me.

"Stop!" The erotic tension breaks and two erections go limp as if doused with arctic water. "Gentlemen, I have to put in my diaphragm."

"It's okay," replies Jeremy with an air of superior knowledge. "We're tantric."

I stare at him in disbelief.

"We won't come inside of you."

The goddess might go for that reassurance but not the flesh-and-blood birthday girl. I put in my diaphragm and contemplate the two geishas waiting. As I finish, they fall on me, smothering my body with a blanket of kisses and long, loving strokes with their tongue.

But the spell has broken. I ache for the gentle, electric caresses I need so much. I am distracted as if there were another person present in the room. It makes me shiver because this presence is both familiar and strange.

I close my eyes and see Fausto bending over me. The expression on his face betrays a jarring blend of jealousy and excitement. He kisses me deeply and I feel like a cold, dormant volcano that has suddenly become active and erupts, spreading a fluid fire clear down to my toes. My body throbs and twists with yearning. Fausto pulls away, smiles and strokes my hair.

I glance at Jeremy and Alexander, who are once again massaging me and seem to be oblivious to Fausto's presence. I close my eyes again and Fausto dissolves me further with another kiss that reaches far into my womb. I am liquid and utterly receptive. He pulls back, savoring my delicious agony. I arch my head, desperate to hold on to his lips.

Don't stop, please!

One more deep electric kiss makes my eyes water and I pant heavily. His mouth slides down my neck to a place he once christened the "hot spot." It is my true Achilles' heel. Fausto is the only man to understand just how much this spot makes me vulnerable, a slave to his passionate touch. He softly bites around this spot, a sensual teasing dance that makes blood surge through my veins, heart pound frantically and every muscle twitch uncontrollably. The rhythm of his lips and teeth on my neck matches that of Alexander's cock, which is now sliding gracefully in and out, in and out of my cunt.

More, more. Anything. Just don't stop.

The combination of sultry Fausto and Alexander is more than I can bear. The steady rhythm of Alexander's cock, now soaring up and out, then in and down—coupled with the memory of Fausto's melodious touch and sizzling kisses—has turned me into an orgasmic butterfly. Each moan and gasp for breath is like the flutter of my wings, lifting me higher, higher and higher still, until I finally soar among the stars, propelled by what seems like cosmic waves. Shivers of pleasure permeate every fiber, pore and crevice in my body.

"Fausto!"

His name reverberates in my mind like a simultaneous shriek and prayer as I break through an excruciating barrier that leaves me limp and drenched in sweat.

# And After I Submit

*UNSIGNED*

I was taking my chances returning to Andre's tiny stucco cottage. As I stood at his door and smelled the roses twining up either side, I recalled our last encounter, two weeks before. I had run out of this same doorway in the wee hours, into pouring rain, frightened and enraged. He had been suddenly furious with me for reasons I little understood. I only knew that it had something to do with his insatiable hungers. These, I was certain, must be nearly as old as he was. I had often seen the enraged four-year-old in him demanding the impossible. I had given it my best and he had taken it all, ruthlessly. The more carefully and precisely I had administered caresses and affections, yieldings and special favors, the more inflamed had become his desire, and the more exacting and cruel his demands. Finally he had exhausted me, mentally and physically.

That last evening I had devoted myself totally to fulfilling his exotic appetites with the most varied of pleasures. But he would not be satisfied. Some demon—some crazy light—had shown through his eyes. It was a look I had seen in him before and it frightened me. It always preceded one of his tempers. It had a quality of desperate fear, a wildness that wrenched my stomach and alerted my senses to ready me for any possibility.

This night the demon would not be soothed. After our lovemaking, I had begged Andre to let me sleep. He became irritable and demanded that I make him come once more. Utterly drained, I hadn't the strength to raise a hand. "Please,"

221

I thought, "Andre, don't let the demon out tonight." The alarm rushing through my body gave me new energy to reach over his back and gently stroke him. "Please, can't we wait till morning, love?" I pleaded. My refusal had the effect of a match to gunpowder. His rage flared, obliterating any remaining tenderness between us. I noticed his arms tensing and bending as he rose to his knees over me. Sensing approaching violence, I surveyed in an instant's glance all possibilities for escape. Now fully alert, I knew I would have to move quickly when the moment came. I softened like a kitten to avoid triggering one of the taut springs in his arms into pinning me down, then I slid out from under him with such smooth precision that my pants, blouse and shoes were on, though not zipped or buttoned, before he came after me. In a single flow of silently efficient speed, I moved to the door and rushed out.

With rain pouring and my heart doing double time, I ran. Not that I feared his pursuit. Months of overindulgence in drugs and alcohol had rendered him no match for my speed. I wanted only to be far away from the demon in him. I ran for nearly half an hour, until I reached the steps of my own apartment. The moment I got the door opened, the phone began to ring. I knew if I answered he would plead, then insist, that I come back. I walked to the phone and, sure of what I wanted, unplugged it. As I turned away from the silenced machine, a stony anger rose in me and hardened my jaw.

Standing in the noon sunlight, faintly aware of a red rose bobbing next to the doorbell, I considered for a moment whether I was making a mistake. I had returned not with any reasonable expectation of rapprochement, but with a primitive sort of longing. In two weeks I had been unable to dismiss the desire for Andre's tenderness and passion. He had stirred me with an intensity I'd never experienced before. With a single look, he knew me completely. His eyes found the very center of my being; perhaps he could see the actual genetic composition of the cells of my body. I was a piece of thread which he drew through the eye of a needle. One of his glances could tell me to follow him, to speak or to join him in play. All his commands and wishes I had obeyed with a willingness that came from inside. My obedience was not willed; it was instinctual. I had come back for more of the exquisite pleasure of being so connected with another human being.

As I raised my arm to press the doorbell, I felt a tingling excitement, a mixture of desire and danger. After a few moments the door opened slowly. Andre stood wordless, motionless, his brown eyes regarding me softly. He was a cherub in the guise of a man, but not too soft. I was grateful for one more occasion to enjoy his physical beauty. His brown hair was curly, almost ringlets but not quite. Any mother would have doted on him (and he'd had plenty of substitutes). His proportions seemed perfectly complementary to my own. Only he was three inches taller than I. And we fit together like two pieces of wet clay.

He seemed to be waiting for me to say why I was there. Receiving no invitation to enter filled me with a slight awkward embarrassment. "May I come in?" I asked. He stepped aside, still not speaking, and I crossed the threshold. I longed for the welcoming embrace I had grown accustomed to. If only he would throw his arms around me and lead me directly to bed. But his arms hung stiffly at his sides. I felt even more awkward, off balance. We stood for a few moments at a tender distance. He seemed to control the boundary between us with his eyes. I was fixed to the spot. I searched his eyes for some sign that he was glad to see me, but found no clue. His regard remained soft but impenetrable. Swallowing my pride, I reached to embrace him. He returned the embrace, perfunctorily. Suddenly I felt stiff and mechanical, like a doll whose joints move back and forth on a single axis. A panic rose in me and I hated myself for having come. "It really is over," I thought. "He has nothing to give me." I searched for magic words to make everything better, the way it used to be. Nothing came. My throat was closing up. Perhaps I could say, "I'm sorry." But sorry for what? There I stood, mute, looking longingly into his eyes, like some devoted pet dog. He continued to survey me with a distant and inscrutable gaze. I wondered how he could remain effortlessly composed. Then, slowly, all promptings quieted inside me. My body eased, and I stood with nothing to say, absolutely still. At that precise moment, he took me by the hand and, with a look, commanded me forward. We walked through his gray front room and into the bedroom. At once I felt tiny and soft, like a child princess. A pleasure filled me like that I had felt long ago on Christmas morning, approaching the tree and the bright packages with my name on them. Gratitude welled up in me for having been forgiven—although for what I did not know.

His bed was unmade, as usual. Diagonal shafts of sunlight sliced across the slightly grayed tangle of covers. He placed his hands on my shoulders from behind and turned me to face him. Holding me at arms' length he moved his hands to my waist and gave me a look that said, "You're here for me," with total assurance of his right to my favors. Like butter, I began to melt. I heard my inner voice saying, "Yes, I am here for you alone." I stood still, knowing he could mold me to his desire. He unbuttoned my blouse. A surge of playful catlike impulses rose through my legs, into my groin and up through the rest of my body. I pulled his shirt out of his pants and down his graceful arms. I loosened his pants and stopped to lower them, feeling vulnerable with my bare ass arching out behind me. The sight of his cock, stiff and slightly curved, aroused me. With practiced ease he stepped out of his trousers. I took his cock in my hand and stroked it, marveling at its suede smoothness.

Again he took my hand in his and raised me up. We went to the narrow bed, straightened the sheets and slid in between. Not that covers were necessary: we fit together face to face so snugly that not an inch of space was left between us for cool air. Embracing thus, noses nearly touching, we looked deep into each other's eyes. Pleasure filled me like warm mist. I felt all the surfaces of my body dissolve as we fused. We were bigger than the room containing us—in a universe without time.

The fucking was as soft as velvet and as hard as finality. He shaped me into a dozen different forms—curved, flat, upright, bent diagonally. He pushed my legs up and back over my head so far I thought my ass would split. His strokes were both hot and cold. I squeezed and pressed into his flesh with my fingers, my teeth sinking as deeply into his shoulder as I dared without drawing blood. Floating, I rebounded from his solidity, bobbing yet anchored to his stiff plump cock. Too soon, a fine layer of perspiration began to cover my body. Limp and taut at once, I felt all the cells of my skin would burst from the tension of the moment. Sensing the instant beyond which I could no longer endure, Andre spoke in a voice insistent and sure. There was a dark tone of threat in it which made my skin tingle. "Come now!" he commanded. And my orgasm came like gusts of tropical rain, cascaded into a thunderous waterfall and pooled off into quiet reflections of sky on smooth water. He allowed me a few long moments to lie still. My mind's eye floated through deep green pools, over their white foam and into thin mists drawn up by the sun. Then I felt his hand move lower on my damp stomach toward my furry patch. He pushed his fingers into the slippery opening and stroked firmly and rhythmically. A jolt ran up my spine like bullets, riveting me for a moment at helpless attention. I arched as the charge spread out from my backbone in every direction. He pulled his fingers out as quickly as he had slid them in, and, tugging at my hips, motioned me to turn over. As soon as I had rolled onto my stomach, he pulled me up onto my knees. He slid underneath me on his stomach and said, "Fuck me." My bones had come to life again. They moved inside my skin. Mounted on his back, I hugged him hard and squeezed his legs together with my thighs. Then with my breasts flush against him, I began thrusting my pelvis over his buttocks, hot as the sand on a sun-soaked beach. I pushed again and again into their cushiony yielding. A physical power took shape in my pelvis, focusing outward, into his ass. Even without a cock, I knew I was fucking him in the ass. I quickened my tempo, feeling more alive with each thrust. I was penetrating him with all the concentrated force of my being. We both began to moan in unison with a spontaneity that made every moment a discovery. My hips were as fluid as mercury. Soon I could contain my excitement no longer. Tears and laughter erupted from every pore. Weakly I collapsed beside him. Andre, still vigilant with appetite, commanded me again, "Fuck me!" I raised myself up onto one elbow and reached for the jar of Vaseline on the floor next to the bed. I opened it and stuck my hand into the cool, gooey gel. To disarm him, with my other hand I stroked his brow and cheek as tenderly as a mother, and then found his bottom with my other hand. Quickly my finger found the opening and pushed in. Andre gave a little yelp of fear and pleasure and squeezed his hole tight against my entrance. His opening was as strong and hot as a cunt. I pushed harder. He opened slowly. As I pushed in and out, he squeezed and opened and squeezed and opened. His ass reached up higher, wanting me deeper. As he opened wider to me, I slipped in a second finger and stretched him more open still. Then a third, and a fourth. Undulating and moaning, his movements quickened. Knowing the moment was near, I pulled out my fingers and turned him onto his side. I slid under him and pulled him tight to me. His body was heavy with surrender. Once inside me, he pumped slowly and powerfully. He came in moments, arching and straightening his back as his hot ejaculate rushed into me. His face gave off soft showers of light, and his voice escaped from deep inside him, high-pitched and helpless. We sank into the mattress, holding each other in sweet muddy embrace.

Our semiconscious reverie seemed endless. In the quiet tender protection of each other's arms, we were children without fear, without memory, whole and new.

We dressed wordlessly. Andre again took me by the hand and led me slowly to the door. We exchanged a last passionate kiss, and I drifted through the door into the sunlight.

# TRANSFORMATION

## *Prisoners*

### *SYN FERGUSON*

When I was very small I heard colors and saw sounds. The sound of my mother's name, Shirley, was a dark maroon-red I thought ugly then. I "watched" music in my head, weaving lines of color that flowed from thin, intense rays to throbbing blushes that spread and faded in the air, colors layered like the petals of flowers or falling like feathers. For the things adults gave no words—like the plastic, folded skin on drying mud—I gave my own until they laughed and said no one would understand me. That laughter hurt, so I learned not to hear the colors, not to see the music. I learned that the pleasure of my white explosion on the edge of sleep was wrong, learned to please others instead of myself.

By the age of five I had mastered living in an arbitrary reality. I shut myself up like a prisoner and became my own guard, and I learned to lie. Since the essence of a lie is to please the listener I learned not to be too colorful, too pleasant or intense. Only a small child would say the dog wet her pants. No, lies must be monochrome, like dreams, to please my listeners. It did not matter that the lies were playful possibilities or that I swam through brilliant storms of neon in my sleep. The prisoner must not send messages in code.

I have read how, in other cultures, the maidens are led down to the riverbank (with garlands and praise) to have the pleasure cut out of them. When the knifework begins, older women who have suffered the same pain chant and sing to drown the screaming. Gifts such as I had run in families. My grandmother dreamed death—her sister playing a piano with black velvet keys, the hired hand digging a well so deep he could not climb out of it. She kept my mother from seeing a motion picture until she was thirteen, and then, when Momma won a talent contest at seventeen, she was afraid to leave her mother and accept the prize. I know who sang while I was silenced.

Having been imprisoned all my life, do you think I should welcome an hour's release that only demonstrates some warden's power? Do the Egyptian dead, millennia safe in their tombs, wish to have their time-cemented wrappings loosed? When I bring frost-scarred weeds into the warmth and humidity of my house do the dry pods split of their own will to show their silk insides and spill the filaments carrying their doomed seeds? Why should I desire to be broken open, lose the face I have so carefully constructed, expose the prisoner afraid to leave her cell? I don't desire it. I don't desire it. Guards can't move me to it. My prisoner speaks to other prisoners only. *Are you alone? Does it still hurt? Do you remember?*

All my life I have rushed from prison to prison, pretending, for safety's sake, to be a guard. One of these prisons was the Air Force, which had the advantage of clearly drawn lines. There anyone of equal rank or lower qualified as a prisoner and compatriot, anyone of superior rank was a guard and the enemy. All of the conversations of the prison yard turn on the superiority of prisoners, of course. Guards like brutish surroundings and bland food. Guards have no loyalties but to themselves. Prisoners are innocent, guards guilty. That was the dark need that brought me there, the crack in the floor of the bottommost cave through which all the light in my life finally filtered and drained away. I never thought of healing the wound; it was all distinctions with me then: light and dark, good and evil, the innocent and the oppressors. . . .

So we were all prisoners in the Air Force, the forty men and four women of my flight in paramedic training school. After the cramped cells and constant torment of basic training, we had a larger enclosure and less attention from the guards. In this relative freedom we sat out the sweet, hot Alabama evenings on the mess hall steps, at the NCO club, under the bushes behind the barracks. In my particular group, most of us had not turned twenty.

Gary Walker was small, quick, and dark, with a slow West Virginia softness in his speech. Officially he was my boyfriend; that is, if any other male than those Gary had approved spoke to me or sat with me at meals in Gary's absence, he took them out behind the motor pool and beat them up. Gary had been made a prisoner by his parents—literally. At four or five he had asked them some questions about sex. "I didn't even know what it *was!*" he would repeat. "How could I have said anything wrong?" His mother shut him in the unlit cellar for a week without blanket or pillow and put his food on the top step, from which he could eat like a dog or go hungry.

He became his own guard when his younger brother was born in a halcyon period. His parents' marriage and finances had stabilized. The second child was welcomed. Gary also loved the favored son. When Tad got in trouble in school or roused their father's anger, Gary would take the blame. "He can't hurt me," he'd tell Tad, "it's okay. I'm made of steel." Punishment was usually the strap, sometimes the grown man's fist. "I used to pretend to be more afraid than I was," Gary said, "so he'd know I was mocking him, and he'd think I wasn't afraid at all."

Kelly Patrick Smith came to the Air Force a prisoner of his

century and the middle class and found it a poor substitute for the French Foreign Legion. He had trouble with his complexion and his love life. One night when his date had gone home with someone else, K. P. walked back to the barracks and paused to meditate under the slow drift of summer stars. When an M. P. pulled up and demanded to know what he thought he was doing, K. P. realized he had stopped in a railroad crossing. "Waiting for a train," he said bitterly—and spent the night in the lockup.

K. P. and I argued and brangled because we shared the same background and education. We dueled in "verse."

> Argument by sex or station
> is a kitchen helper's ration.
> If needles give you so much pain,
> from charging ladies please refrain.

K. P. set me a valuable example of dealing with the military. They wouldn't *let* you out, but they might *cast* you out. When he skied down the barracks steps and broke his ankle, they gave him a mental discharge.

My attitude was wrong from the first. At my first inspection a sergeant found the beautiful lingerie my mother had provided, "so I would remember I was a woman under the uniform," and *books* in my locker. It finally took a colonel to resolve the problem. I was allowed to keep the underthings if I didn't wear them during duty hours. I kept three books.

The Hungarian brothers were something else. Their last name was Kacsoh. Bela, the elder, must have been in his thirties. He was balding under his crewcut, shrewd, good-tempered and strong. Although he was no taller than I was, Bela could crouch under two floating girls in the pool, put a hand in the small of their backs and raise them up over his own head. He was thick, sleek and rounded, exuding a muscular vitality not subject to fatigue. Condemned to do pushups for some misdemeanor, Bela would do them one-handed or continue until his tormentor was bored with watching.

Though Bela was soundly on the side of the oppressed, he did not experience the amazement at injustice the rest of us did. When his C.O. rescued condemned paint from the dump and kept Bela's whole barracks in from a weekend liberty to paint their equally condemned building, Bela shrugged, organized a work party and had the job done by Saturday noon. When they lost the liberty anyway, for being "too smart," he shrugged again and settled into the air-conditioned NCO club to drink beer. He didn't expect justice from the military, all he wanted was an opportunity to go where Communists were and kill them.

Paul was the younger brother, the only other survivor of the entire family of mother, father, two daughters, four sons. He looked nothing like Bela. In our group Paul was tallest, Bela shortest. Bela was one toast-tan color, his eyes light brown, his hair sandy. Paul was an olive-skinned blond whose dark brows, lashes and beard made a startling contrast against his skin. Paul seldom looked anyone but Bela in the eye; when he did, his eyes were cool gray-green like shadowed water. Instead of Bela's round, open eye, Paul's eyes were deeply set guarded triangles. He always looked a little ashamed, a little afraid. It was a commonplace that if our group was to be censured, it would be Paul who was singled out or put on report.

Bela never defended Paul overtly, but there was a tension in him like the watchful assessment of a sheep dog. Although Paul made a handy butt in the barracks because he was gullible, obedient and he never retaliated, the aimless hazing never went too far. If Paul resented being called a dummy or thought one, he never said so. He seldom spoke at all, and his English was slow and broken. Bela would not tolerate the use of Hungarian among people who could not understand it.

"If you want to be heard, speak English," he said. Paul could not do that, so he stayed silent. What Bela said was law to his brother, although, watching, I sometimes saw color rise in Paul's cheeks at some brusque comment. Once, when Bela broke his own rule and rattled out a harsh Hungarian phrase of correction, I saw a liquid gleam in Paul's eye and an infinitesimal swelling and reddening of the delicate skin of his eyelid. Paul's face did not change at all, then or when I pressed a sympathetic knee against his under the table, but his thigh was so tense it was like touching stone.

Gary, K.P. and I were loungers—staying cool, looking on at life. Bela and Paul were doers, with a brand of physical competency I'd never been exposed to before. Once, when their football lodged in the gutter of the barracks a story and a half above ground level, Bela made a stirrup, Paul stepped from Bela's hands to his shoulders, stretched up and retrieved the ball. When Bela accepted it and strolled casually away from the building, Paul balanced for a long moment and dismounted like a gymnast, with a forward somersault. Both of them could turn flips and walk on their hands, but when I asked what they had done in Hungary, Bela said they had both been students. Their father was a pharmacist.

Paul deferred to everyone, although in a lesser degree than he did to Bela. He stood when there were not enough seats to go around, took the fifth, awkward, place at a table designed for four, and always drew the chair farthest from me at a dance. He seemed to accept Gary's rights of ownership and seldom looked directly at me, but once or twice at each dance, Paul would silently approach and hold out his hand. As we danced he would slowly and inexorably draw me closer and closer until my leg was trapped between his legs, his leg moving between mine, and I was pressed against him from thigh to breast. Slowly, and with no change in his face, he would grind his hard erection against my belly or my thigh for the duration of the dance. I neither protested nor reciprocated. I never stopped dancing or became aroused myself. I suppose my face was as blank as his. Certainly I never felt the exchange had anything to do with Gary. In a way they were equally inexplicable to me—Gary's jealousy and Paul's physical response.

Since he had never objected to my dancing with Paul before, I think the fight happened because someone else made a comment to Gary. It happened at the one party Bela did not attend, and after someone had spiked the punch. It was one of those hot nights. We were too broke to buy beer at the end of the pay period, and thirsty. These company-sponsored bashes offered the only entertainment on base: a band and a dance floor, free soft drinks, game tables for cards, chess and Scrabble. Gary usually didn't drink hard liquor, and the potency of the punch came as a surprise, but having poured, he had to drink, and drink again to prove the first time had not been an accident. It muddled him enough to throw off his chess game, and I was standing behind him when he lost. There was a moment of confusion and embarrassment while Gary, fogged by alcohol, couldn't see the checkmate until his opponent actually moved the piece and took his king. Gary hated to be shown up or laughed at; I drifted back to the dance floor. I have forgotten who I was with when K.P. cut in to tell me that Gary and Paul were fighting.

"Fighting?" I couldn't believe it. Gary had approved Paul, and Paul did not fight. I followed K.P. outside.

A white flurry of moths were battering themselves against

a floodlight and under it a dozen people had gathered around two straining, slipping bodies. If you give CPR and have seen it pantomimed, you know the difference between a stage fight and a real one. Gary was trying to kill Paul, to tear off an ear, gouge out an eye, kick his balls or beat his head against the brick building. He was flushed and panting with his efforts to get a permanent hold and twist something off; Paul was white and desperate. There were men in that crowd bigger and stronger than Gary. They believed that Paul was retarded, but none of them opened a way for him to escape. When Gary knocked Paul into the circle of watchers, they would move back enough to let him fall. When he did, Gary was right there with his spit-shined shoes, kicking and stamping at Paul's face.

"Get the M.P.s," I yelled at K.P., my voice as useless as a whistle in a paper bag. He nodded to show he understood me, but even as he went, his face was turned back toward the fight, where Gary went on and on, with boundless energy in the blood-warm air, trying to kill Paul.

When the M.P.s did come, finally, Paul was on his knees, arms raised overhead, while Gary smashed blow after blow at him with both hands. It wasn't the blood or the sound that was so shocking, but the fact that Gary was so obviously trying to erase the fact of Paul's existence with his bare hands.

He didn't see or hear the M.P.s. It took a nightstick, swung with savage force against the back of his thighs, to make him look up from his attack. As he turned to see what had hurt him, the hilt of the second nightstick hit his temple and he went slowly to his knees and then much faster, totally limp, down on his face.

We were in Alabama for medical training. Nothing I learned in class ever made a deeper impression than the confidence that M.P. had in the thickness of Gary's skull.

With Paul bleeding on his knees and Gary unconscious, I
started forward. The M.P. barred my way with his stick
across my middle. He didn't hit me with it, barely touched
me. There was no need for K.P. to screech hysterically in
his face.

The M.P. took out a notebook, and the bystanders, who
were still looking almost enviously at Gary's sprawled form
and Paul gasping for air, began to drop back into the shadows. Nobody knew why the fight had started. Nobody knew
anything. The M.P. took down names and serial numbers
while Gary lay unconscious and Paul bled. They would not
call an ambulance, would not get a doctor.

The next morning we learned from Bela that both Paul and
Gary had finally been examined. Gary had been taken to the
hospital to have his right hand put in a cast, and Paul was
being given the maximum administrative punishment for fighting: fifteen days in the stockade. This was not the overnight
lockup on our small training base, but a real military prison at
nearby Maxwell Field. Bela said he was going AWOL to try
to see Paul. He did hitchhike to Maxwell but was picked up
by the M.P.s and did not see his brother. Then he was confined
to barracks, like Gary.

For the next week, K.P. and I became pariahs. No one moved
in to usurp Gary's rights because Gary had half killed Paul,
who stood a foot taller and outweighed him fifty pounds. And
*no one* spoke up for Paul, although half our flight had been
present and seen Gary trying to kill him. I could not reconcile
my feelings. I still woke up at night, aching for Gary, wanting
him, but when I finally saw him, an actual physical sensation
of cold spread from my center outward. He walked into the
mess hall at dinnertime, after K.P. and I had been through the
line. The cast got in his way and he had trouble managing his
tray. K.P. made a half-movement to get up and help Gary, and

as he did, I swept my tray off the table and left. The next morning, after a night when I woke myself up crying, K. P. and Gary walked together toward my table, but I got up and moved away. After that we didn't speak. Bela was released, and he and I now formed a defensive alliance.

I suppose it was worse for Bela. He and Gary had to sleep in the same dormitory, share the same shower, sweat next to each other in formation. I merely sat in the same classroom, but I can still remember the feeling of being caught up and twisted in slow, electric currents. The whole flight was affected. Rowdy horseplay gave way to whispered but emphatic credos. Bela and I didn't hear these comments, but they had to do with Paul, and they were ugly and unfair—or why would we have felt so defensive, so beleaguered?

There is nothing like misery accompanied by heat, humidity and the cloying lemon-vanilla sweetness of magnolia. Night after night I would lie naked under my sheet, wanting Gary, my mind ringed by white circles of thought like those moths streaking and curving around the floodlight. Every flight came to an abrupt halt against the white, burning barrier of injustice. No more than those moths could I escape the one fact that was hurting me. Gary's anger had hurt Paul, who hurt no one. Even if I were marginally willing to grant the existence of an anger out of control, it had cooled eventually, and Gary still let Paul take the blame. "How could she do it?" Gary had asked me over and over of his mother. How could she lock an innocent child in the basement for a week and feed him like a dog? How could Gary do it? I wondered through the nights. In the morning there were never any answers, only the dry husks and charred wings, an ashy residue of thought.

Paul was released on a Saturday. Bela and I planned a picnic for him; that is, Bela borrowed a friend's car, got permission to use another friend's summer place in the country, purchased the food and set up the schedule. All I had to do was be decorative. I put on a dress I had bought with Gary in mind. It was a leaf-green shirtwaist with a full skirt and a belt made of three grosgrain ribbons: rose, lavender and blue. Under the dress I wore the forbidden lingerie my mother had provided, pale green, the full half slip three tiers of ruffles.

Paul was in uniform when we picked him up, his face not just blank but closed. He climbed in the back seat of the car and didn't comment on my dress or the picnic basket. He didn't ask where we were going. Bela drove in a determined silence, and I had momentary fantasies that we were going AWOL, fleeing the country, escaping somehow. Instead we drove gradually rising roads, climbing into a cooler, prettier country. We turned onto a dusty private road and parked the car beside a boarded-up cabin. Bela took the picnic basket and the blanket and led the way past the cabin and across a field dotted with Queen Anne's lace to a stand of cottonwoods. We stepped over a slack, curling strand of barbed wire, ducked under a branch and stood in cool, green gloom. A shimmer of silver-green winked at us between the gray-brown trunks, and drifts of floss floored the wood. The undersides of the still leaves were silver. The trees made a circle around a pond choked with green growth. Bela led the way to a sloping lawn where people had camped and cooked before. There was a ring of stones, an iron spit for barbecuing.

We were awkward with each other. Paul's silence had infected me. Bela spread his blanket and settled his champagne in a plastic bag of ice while Paul and I watched. "I'm going in," he said, and stripped to his swimming trunks and plunged into the water. His walrus thrashing shattered the oppressive silence and set the whole pond rocking and winking with light. Floating clouds of cottonwood floss drifted toward the reeds. I took off my shoes and began to wade. The water was only pleasantly cool, and the silt underfoot was soft as velvet.

"Come on," I told Paul. "It's great."

He shook his head a little, looked for Bela, and saw that he was facedown and splashing. "I have not brought—" He had only the clothes he'd gone to the stockade in, of course. I hadn't thought about their being the same ones.

"Wear your shorts. There's nobody here but us." I turned back to my wading. If Paul swam I wouldn't have to make conversation. I was indifferent to his state of dress. It was Gary's small, muscled tightness I wanted. I wandered down the bank. After a while I heard the splashing increase. Paul and Bela were trying to drown each other. My misery lifted a little. I found a place where the bottom slanted toward a miniature forest of swaying waterweed. I stepped down to feel the feathery strands with my feet and slid deeper than I'd intended. When I tried to climb back I couldn't get traction.

Bela came to the rescue, or so I thought. Exercise, or the fact that Paul had joined him at it, had filled him with the spirit of mischief. Instead of helping me, he reached out and unfastened the top button of my dress.

"Bela!" I retreated, holding up my skirts.

He took a step deeper, reaching for another button. I turned sideways. Bela pretended to look under my skirt. Paul approached through the swaying weeds.

"Bela, if you ruin this dress—"

He denied the possibility and unfastened another button. He said he would hang the dress up for me. I said like hell he would. Bela tethered me by the ribbons at my waist and told Paul they were going to have their will with me. Paul glided closer and reached for my wrists under the froth and flutter where I clutched skirt and slip. His cool hands cradled my wrists, never closing over them. For that reason, and on behalf of the sea-green underwear, I let Bela make an elaborate production out of unbuttoning my dress, untying the ribbons, taking the pins from my hair. Finally the half slip had to come off over my head, and while they were occupied with keeping everything dry, I dived between them and swam away. Bela threatened Hungarian revenge while he hung my things over a branch. Paul just stood in the water looking after me.

It felt good to be cool all over and swim hard. Bela declared a mermaid sighting and we played tag around the pond. One moment Paul would be plunging and splashing with us, his water-cooled thigh grazing mine, or his fingers lightly closing and releasing around my ankle; the next he would be floating by himself, passive and focused inward while his white body sank down through the lily-green water. When he sighed and waded for shore, Bela gave me an apologetic look and followed him.

From my feathery entanglement with another underwater garden, I watched the two brothers talking, and my mood sank down to match Paul's. Why was it so hard to be happy? Bela only wanted Paul to thrive in his new country. I only wanted Gary to be fair so I could comfort him again.

Idly I let them drift out of focus, out of the present. Against that tapestry of varied green they looked like figures from legend, from fairy tales. Bela's barrel body and massive shoulders suited the ill-formed dwarf who shoed the horses, scrubbed the pots, polished the armor. Beside him Paul was tall and fair, crowned with gold and despair. Bela reached out and touched Paul's arm in a comforting gesture, but Paul jerked back. His voice rose, the pain clear through the language barrier. At the end of his speech he slammed his fist into his groin and made a shocking, savage gesture of throwing away. Bela stepped back. Paul turned and flung himself facedown on the blanket. He said something that cut Bela like a knife. My heart was thumping. I didn't understand what was happening, but it broke the pattern. Paul always obeyed Bela. Bela always knew what to do.

It was clear that he didn't know now. He took an uncertain step toward the blanket, then drew back and came toward the pond.

I went to meet him. "What's wrong?"

Bela walked past me to stand waist-deep in the water. He took two deep breaths. "Always since the Communists come, things happen. There are deaths. We have hard times. Lose everything. Not my fault, not Paul's, no one but those godless pigs— Never in my life will I forget, but I will *have* no life if I remember all day, each day. Paul remembers, all the time. He feels much guilt. He cannot be happy." Bela slapped a great blade of glittering spray out of the water. It fell back, silver into green, and was gone again.

His shoulders slumped. "Tibor was nine and Paul was thirteen. We left them safe, in a basement, while we scout the frontier. The food was bad; they were cold, sick. Tibor died. What should Paul have done with no medicine, no weapon, too sick to walk? If I had been a man, he tells me. They were children. It is no shame on him. Now *this* happens. How can it be his fault there are"—harsh foreign word—"in the world?"

I made him explain. It's an old story in prisons. Paul had drawn eyes with his height and fairness. His passiveness and depression were taken for another kind of docility. The attack had stopped short of rape, but the only protection had been solitary confinement, a prison within a prison.

"He liked you," Bela said, as if he were talking about some third person not present. "He tells me how soft your skin, how your waist moves, that your hair shines in the sun. You fire his blood, and I am happy because—I speak frankly—we have been alone together too long. Paul makes no friends. In the camps he was still a child. We lived on lemonade and potatoes.

Even I did not think of women. Here we eat, he grows—like a weed, like a tree—taller than me. Like a prince he is beautiful, and he feels his— He feels he is a man, but he cannot speak! Still he has no one but me.

"We please each other," Bela said bluntly. "It is easy for me, a kindness for one I love. Brothers do this. Does it change that I am a man for women? No. That he is? No and no!

"Now this filth, these rumors. Again he blames himself. I can't help him!" He struck the water again.

Tears and a kind of weariness stung my eyes as I watched the reflection shift and sway. Bela could not help Paul, whom he loved. I could not help Gary. And I was there, cool as pond water in my now transparent underthings. There had always been a pleasant sexual tension between Bela and me. Thoughts skimmed the surface of my mind like dragonflies. Men put so much meaning in sex. What difference does the body make when the self has all those catacombs to hide in? What was faithfulness? Rules? Or setting right what Gary had indirectly precipitated? Could it be set right? Prisoners have to help each other.

We went to the blanket together and knelt on each side of Paul. He stiffened when he heard us and flinched when Bela touched him. Wordlessly I followed Bela's lead in a slow, stroking massage down Paul's body. It was a good body, long, strong, graceful, the skin smooth, the flesh warm and firm. It carried a salty tang of perspiration and a sweet breath of pond water. I matched Bela's strokes, giving my hands and strength to the work, faintly envying the fact that touching came easy for him. Bela was always steadying, guiding, patting, caressing—or elbowing, tackling, pushing, punching.

He didn't stop at Paul's waist, even though Paul wasn't relaxing. Under the wet white cotton Paul's buttocks were set like stone. "Lift up," Bela commanded, peeling the wet briefs

down. Under my palms I felt Paul's protest and then the slight
yielding that let Bela slide the fabric down his legs. My hands
kept working, cooperating with Bela's. A hollowness was growing in me, an empty space I had to breathe deeply to fill.

Bela looked at me. *Who are you, stranger? Prisoner or guard?*

I nodded and he pulled his swimming trunks off and tossed
them after Paul's briefs. Disconnected, my mind revolved around
two questions I had considered before. How is it that men
look so long without that line at the waist? and why does the
smooth head of a man's penis always make me conscious that
it is so much the texture of my own lips—a special, sensitive
flesh?

Without words, Bela's hands showed me how beautiful, how
long, strong and praiseworthy Paul was. He added kisses to
his stroking, and after a moment I followed, safely above the
waist at first, then to the small of the back, which made the
spine arch and sink in, to the side where the sensitive flesh
shivered and shrank away. The skin on Paul's ass was smooth
under my lips. Bela's head bumped mine and he grinned at
me, a little sheepishly. I saw that his cock was stretching and
thickening as we worked on Paul. It was such an awkward
protrusion from his body, now prodding Paul's back or thigh,
next grazing the back of my hand like a scrap of velvet. Always
bumping into things, I thought giddily. Perhaps it was the
shortage of air.

Paul rolled over, finally, yielding to our urging. His head
was turned toward Bela; he had clenched his hands into fists,
thrown his arm over his eyes. His chest was smooth, but the
hair under his arms and round his cock was dark, like his
eyelashes and his beard. It made him look shockingly naked,
shockingly male. Bela leaned forward and kissed his lips. I
followed his example. Paul kissed like a child. The faint, returning pressure of his lips came almost too late. I slid down

his chest with kisses, following Bela. Pulses beat at odd points in my body—inside my elbow, behind my knee, fluttering in my side. I saw Bela draw a circle around Paul's nipple with his tongue and a pang shot through me. My own nipples stood up hard.

Bela turned his head and saw. He reached across Paul, took my shoulders and bent to kiss me through the fabric of my bra, making an instant fire between my legs. The hollowness spread. Paul uncovered his eyes to watch as Bela fumbled with the hooks and eyes of my bra, pulling my hair a little in the process. The bra snapped open, and Bela pulled back, sliding the straps down my arms, pulling the adhesive lace free. He bent and sucked my nipple into his mouth. I arched toward him, my spine tensing of itself into a strychnine curve that would throw me over and back and open. Between us, Paul's cock twitched and began to grow. My left breast was abandoned in air until Paul reached up and touched it, a whisper of fingertips against skin.

These things the body manages best by itself, the little heat, the hollowness becoming intention. That's all right, do it without me, I'll be back when you're through. Bela's hands were urging me out of my underpants and astride, pumping Paul with a knowing hand like a master mechanic: turn this, oil that, press here. He stroked me open and went with the head of Paul's cock, then found the channel. Now he was Dr. Kildare, delivering the baby. You're all right, you're all right. Everything's going to be fine, one more big one now, PUSH!

Paul slid into me, but he was insecure, only half hard and ready to withdraw. I thought how pointless and awkward this was, like drinking and posing for strangers you don't care to impress at a party you don't want to attend. We both froze, Paul and I. Only Bela, sweating and anxious, was still heated. The bitch in me, the uniformed matron, said, oh, well, trade partners, at least he's a man. Get yours and to hell with the prisoner.

Totally inappropriate thought at a totally inappropriate time. Why can't Gary see who that voice *is?* Why can't he see why it separates us? That I hate the guard, I will die a prisoner before I become one?

As if the thought had been transmitted through the flesh, Paul said, "Gary—"

The skin on my breasts and belly crawled, trying not to be naked, not to be joined to Paul, not to have Bela's hand steadying my back, his glistening fist hovering over Paul's stomach.

"Gary told them," Paul said, his English hesitant, but his voice firm.

"What?" My hair was falling in my eyes, but the gesture to put it right was only worn with clothes. If I moved I would only dislodge Paul or feel him more, as I felt and resented Bela's comforting strokes on my back.

"He told them," Paul insisted. "He told them he made the fight."

"When?" After he was safe, I thought. After he saw how I treated him.

"The same night—" a quick spill of Hungarian.

"Speak English," Bela said, still the mentor.

"When he had not anger," Paul said. "The first night."

A heated flood of feeling rose up and spilled out of my eyes. There were tears in Paul's green eyes, tears between Bela's cheek and my shoulder, the tears that prisoners weep, wishing for freedom. Paul slid out of me and pulled me down. We all lay down on the blanket, a huddle of arms and legs and flowing emotion, comforting each other. At last Bela brought napkins from the picnic basket. I blew my nose.

"Why didn't they let you go?" I asked Paul.

"It matters not," Paul said. "He had you to go to. I am not even a man."

Bela and I both reached for him.

"You *are* a man," Bela corrected. "A man may weep, a man may grow weary, and fail, and still be a man. Much has been taken from you, but this no one can take. Little son, little prince, you *are* a man."

Languorously, Bela stroked down Paul's side, then down mine. He looked at his palm as if he could read the future there. Tear-stained, the two of us watched him think, students to his teacher.

"Here." He knelt up and urged me to sit in his lap, lean back against his muscular body. His hands cupped my buttocks a moment, then slid under to my thighs. With his effortless strength he lifted me, doubling me back on myself, opening me. I could feel myself parting like the sections of an orange. Paul knelt, too, his face still marked with tears, his wet lashes in starry points. His cock was hardening and lifting, darkening to that evening-rose color that throbs like the deepest organ note. I heard it with my ears, my teeth, my bones. The vibration shook all of us, stronger, deeper, as he found his place. The same note filled the hollowness, a bone-shaking drone that never altered as he pushed in and in. Above and behind him the leaves were willowgreen, amber, translucent jade, sounds open and lonely as flutes and oboes. A bird sang and the notes fell down like flakes of fire.

There was no effort, no shock. Bela's strength absorbed it, his cock, crushed between my hip and his belly, throbbed back after each stroke, *again, again,* as Paul drove through me toward his brother's body. No fear now that the distant light was a trick or a lure. This door would not slam as I approached it. An enchantment of color and sound was laid down before me.

My blood scalded me as I was carried up and up the tunnel, farther out into brightness. FREE.

FREE.

FREE.

And falling as Paul fell back, Bela unfolded me to rest on Paul. Breathing, waiting while we breathed. Paul's face was full of wonder, his belly trembling under my hand, his ribs lifting and lifting to draw in air. He put his hands on my back to feel my heart trying to beat free. Bela knelt over us, unreleased, his cock still tight and dry, just grazing my wet moss. How strong he had been. How kind. I smiled at Paul and raised my hips.

In one long slide, Bela was in me, pointing down, through me, at Paul. We held still, feeling the aftershocks from Paul, the salty foam he'd pumped into me. Bela's hands drew my hips higher, and I rested my forehead on Paul's belly. What an intelligent, curious cock Bela had. *Here? This way? Like that?*

Paul's tired cock stirred to hear my answer.

These are the words written in flesh. We spoke them cock to cunt without memory of past or fear of future:

*You are my target, I your arrow.*

*Oh, wound me, wound me.*

Thick greasy sliding on that pole of meat. Paul soft velvet-satin skin to my lips, Bela rasping like sharkskin inside me. My lips swollen, my throat raw, every pore of my body opened like a floodgate.

*More, yes, more, there. Oh, there!*

Drawing in, gathering. Gold under pressure blurs, flows—molten—ignited. *You are, I am, we become rivers of fiery gold. Who would run, who would hide from such bright destruction?*

Paul arched up, ramming my mound, Bela's balls, quenching us, coming with us in a liquid outpouring of love.

We made love.

The three of us together.

Fell down again, burst of gold, glitter of song, not quite sure where one began and the other ended.

Bela poured wine and peeled ripe peaches from his picnic basket. A rosy flush went through the golden flesh to the red stone, and for a moment I thought I heard how that color sounded. Then it was gone. He fed us with his fingers, and the sweet juice dripped like honey. We smiled and didn't speak and took the last of the wine and stood in the green water drinking it. We bathed each other.

When it was time to go, dressing had become an unfamiliar ritual. It felt wrong to put on so many layers between us: soft cotton of Paul's briefs, cool smoothness of his silvertans. The brothers kissed me into my clothes, marveling at the number of fastenings: hooks, eyes, elastic. Paul lifted my green slip and dropped it down again to see the ruffles flare out. They watched while I combed and pinned my hair. Paul held my dress for me like a coat. Bela buttoned the buttons and knotted the ribbons, each in its proper place where I had creased it before.

He trailed the streamers through his hand, rose, lavender, blue. Let them fall. "No one would ever know they had been untied."

Secrets, I thought, are like the prisoner, reaching through the bars: *Let me out, Let me out.* Silence is what remains when the guard has gone home and the prisoner gone free.

# The Growing Season

## JACQUIE ROBB

Dear Nancy,

I miss you! As the weeks go by, and your letters contain only exterior, surface impressions of your life, I'm frustrated, missing the special contact we've had. I hope your idea of getting away is working and that you and Frank are feeling close. What's happening? You know my feelings on the subject; nevertheless, I hope you are getting what you want.

Remember walking to our "think rock" the day before you left? The wind was up, making whitecaps on the bay. You told me this trip was your last effort to patch things up with Frank. You sounded so resigned I could have cried, even as I gave you reassurance. We sat, not touching, letting the sound of the tide wash through us, the sun warm us. The calm that always enters me in that place finally came, yet I was worried.

It's taken me a while to figure out why I felt both peaceful and unsettled. It's because I wasn't being completely honest with you, or with myself. I'm so slow sometimes! Yes, I wanted to comfort you; of course, I wished you the best. I also wanted to tell you not to go away. If you and Frank can't work it out here, at home on this beautiful Maine coast, what makes you think going back to Ann Arbor is going to do it?

Well, your going away has helped me, if not your marriage. It's helped me clarify my feelings; and being open, even in a letter, even when it bewilders, is better than being dishonest to myself. When you come back ...ah, when you come back...Nan, we've known each other so long; how many times have we cried on each other's shoulders? Laughed together? Brought each other our insights like new toys? How can I help but love you?

So—my feelings for you have grown, my dear, are no longer platonic. I'm in love with you. There, I've said it. I hope this is better than springing

*it on you after you're home. Have your arguments ready ... or your arms
open. My heart is open to you either way.*

*Will we really be seeing each other in only one more month? I can't
wait!*

*Love,*
*Jackie*

*P.S. Don't be scared, just come back. I promise it's safe.*

Two weeks later she still hadn't written in answer. I could
have kicked myself for sending that letter, was kicking myself
for falling in love with a straight woman. And my best friend
at that! I wasn't even listening to my own advice anymore.
Good friends are hard to find, take years of cultivation. Why
throw it all away by falling in love, which, if it doesn't repel
outright, is sure to put strains on the relationship?

Nancy followed my few love affairs at a safe distance as I
was witness for her marriage. She shared my joy and pain with
the same aplomb she carried into her own stormy relationship.
She had always accepted my lesbianism; but acceptance, approval and understanding, I was becoming increasingly aware,
each carried very different emotions.

Somewhere in the back of my mind I knew that our relationship would weather even this turn of events. However,
that didn't keep me from the midnight questions, lying in my
bed upstairs and tracing the patterns of the quilt in the moonlight: Have I scared her off? Will she come to see me? (Oh,
yes. This town just isn't that big.) Will all her defenses be
raised? How can I convince her that it's okay. Whatever happens, it's okay?

I was washing vegetables from the garden, my fingers growing cold under the faucet. The sun was still warm, but the
wind through the screened window was reminding me of all

the chores of autumn. It was almost time for the early radio
news when through the door burst Nancy.

"Wonderwoman!" she cried, her favorite nickname for me.
In one hand was a bunch of devil's paintbrushes and goldenrod.

My whole body warmed as, with wet hands and a gasp, I
hugged her and the bouquet with a bear hug.

"Oh, Nancy, welcome home! When did you get here?"

"Just yesterday. I would have come over sooner, but there
were animals to be soothed...unpacking...you know." Her
tanned face was a healthy highlight for her blond, windswept
hair.

"How's Frank?" I asked, so happy to see her again I could
forgive her her long silence, could even be hopeful for the
reconciliation trip that had separated us.

"In Ann Arbor. Oh, how wonderful everything looks. I'm
so glad to be home," she answered rapidly.

"Then you're really leaving him?" I was too surprised to hide
my excitement. At the same time, my inner voice was telling
me to take the out she had left me.

Her blue eyes darted around my kitchen, looked out the
window and across the fields. "Oh, I don't know. He'll be
visiting his folks for a few weeks, then we'll see."

See what? I wanted to ask, but this time I did hold it back.

I filled a jar with water for the flowers and put the teakettle
on. We settled in at the kitchen table and soon caught each
other up to date. Ann Arbor was certainly not Maine, she said.
Frank had his old school friends to associate with, but their
wives were suburbanites interested in schools, painting classes
and the newest mall going up outside of town. The gleam I
recognized so well came into her eyes as she described, in
hilarious detail, a dinner party at which Frank had discoursed,
in his best academic voice, on the joys of rural living. Nancy,
meanwhile, had sat by, thinking of impenetrable sod, killing

frosts, potato bugs and the spring rains that seemed to hold off each year until the sprouts were at their most vulnerable, requiring all the yearly gained skill and care to salvage. We laughed as we recounted our first discouragements with the wonders of farming. At the back of my mind, though, I was bothered that Nancy still favored Frank as the butt of her jokes.

I was just assuring myself that to have Nancy's wicked wisdom back at the price of silence wasn't so bad when she said:

"I did make friends there, though. Actually, a couple." Her large hands moved to her lap, as if she was suddenly conscious of them.

"Good. Who are they? What are they like?"

"They are lesbians, actually."

"Oh."

"Needless to say, I talked about you a lot."

"Oh."

"I asked them a lot of questions, the questions I was too embarrassed ever to ask you. Or too far away."

"Nancy, listen, I—"

"You're my best friend, Jackie, remember? I suppose I'm flattered about the way you feel about me. Confused, but flattered."

"Well, and what did your friends tell you about me?" I was caught off guard and felt defensive.

"They told me I ought to be talking to you," she replied quietly.

I held out my rough, calloused hand to her; she hesitated just a moment before giving me hers. We looked at each other a long time, while outside the anticipation of twilight gathered. She did look confused, and I tried to meet her gaze with all the love and support I felt.

I saved her having to break off first. "Help me cook supper?" I asked gently.

She looked over to the sink, where the afternoon's chore lay unfinished. "Vegetable stew coming up," she smiled.

I left her cutting up broccoli and went out to the shed for an armload of wood. Looking east over the bay and the growing dusk, I let my breath come slowly and deeply. I remembered again the confusion I had thought would last forever when I had asked myself impatiently what it was that I wanted, not yet realizing that the men's arms to which I had reached for comfort could not comfort me the way I desired. I remembered my surprise when I fell in love for the first time. But of course! How simple! It's a woman I desire. Surprise and delight have replaced confusion to this day; yet I never forgot, never allowed myself to forget, the confusion and the hurt.

Nancy seemed to sense my affirmation when I came back and started the kindling in the cookstove.

"Probably every woman I know has thought about sleeping with another woman," she said, continuing aloud her internal dialogue. "Not that they'd tell their husbands or boyfriends, of course. I know I get my emotional support from my women friends. I think that's normal. It's just... well..."

"So try it!" I tried to keep the tone light, but the joke fell flat. A silence followed, at once accusing and awkward.

"Look, I'm not trying to talk you into anything. Let's leave it alone for a while, okay?" I pleaded. I'm sorry I wrote you that letter, I thought. This is something nobody can figure out for you.

I dumped the vegetables in a pot with some water and started to set the table. We waited for the tension to clear. God, we knew each other so well. We sighed simultaneously, smiled to each other sheepishly.

"Let's walk to the point." Nancy seemed surprised at her own suggestion.

"All right." I chucked a few pieces of wood in the stove,

adjusted the dampers and stuck the bubbling stew on a back burner.

"It's getting chilly out these nights." I reached for a sweater.

"If you can't stand winter, you don't deserve summer." An old joke, and harmony was restored.

We set out at a brisk pace, Nancy leading the way on the path through the semidarkness. Would she turn at the think rock? No, she continued down to the right, through the field and into a grove of scraggly pines leaning far out over the cove, clinging to the bit of soil not torn away by storm or erosion. She left me behind in her haste to meet the sea, out to the very end of the point. I remembered that she had spent the summer in the Midwest, away from the ocean that was so much a part of our lives, and I slowed, as much to give her the space to greet an old friend as for the pleasure of watching her silhouette against the backdrop of trees, rocks and bay.

We stood, suspended in time and space, and watched a waxing moon rise from the indigo horizon. No words were needed here. I loved this woman utterly and completely. I would not want to change her in any way.

Finally, Nancy turned and walked back to me, waiting at the edge of the grove. She put her hands on my shoulders, scanning my face with her clear blue eyes. I had trouble meeting her intensity, having so recently calmed my whirl of emotions to the ocean's night calm.

"Jackie, do you know I love you?"

"Yes, Nancy, I know."

"Will you make love with me, O woman of wonder?"

A pause, the length of a breath, and this time I searched her eyes with my unasked questions.

"Nancy, you don't have to. I—"

"I want to."

"Isn't this something that's just supposed to happen? Spontaneous passion and all that? I don't want you to force yourself because you think this is what I want."

"Isn't that a romantic heterosexist idea?" she teased.

"No, it's not," I replied shortly.

"Okay, okay, I'm open. As an experiment then."

"I am not an experiment."

I watched her read the emotions I was unable to conceal. Then, smiling enigmatically, Nancy leaned forward and kissed me, tentatively, slowly. And I, stunned, then with a leap in my heart of pure anguished joy, enveloped her in my arms. With short tender kisses we explored the boundaries of intimacy. I traced the circle of her mouth with my tongue as her hands stroked my head, ran down my backbone. I searched the face I knew so well, but found it closed to me. I questioned briefly, then let it pass.

Our tension was now of a different, more urgent sort. We shivered with excitement and cold, rubbed each other's arms for warmth and contact, watching our breath crystallize in the night. The mudflats, exposed by the low tide, sent me a pungent, sexual message. The moon's reflection on the water seemed to sanction our connection, haloing our embrace. Our arms around each other, we made our way slowly back to the house.

Wood warmth softened us as we rubbed our hands over the stove's heat.

"It'll be cold upstairs."

"Not for long."

Nancy filled the firebox and put the untouched stew in the warmer while I lit a lamp. Even this momentary separation was too long, and I reached to hold her tightly. Hand in hand, we climbed the stairs.

The moon's silver rays mingled with the lamp's glow as we faced each other. The bureau mirror reflected our profiles in the light: I was just slightly taller than Nancy, with the same, solid build. My short, brown hair contrasted with Nancy's blond mane.

My hand on the top button of her flannel shirt brought her eyes quickly back to mine.

"You are beautiful," I said, bending to kiss what each loosened button revealed. I swept her hair off her face tenderly and her shirt off her shoulders. I let my hands wander over her naked back and waist.

She moved her hands up my sides; I raised my arms and was soon free of my turtleneck. We embraced; breast pressed against breast, belly against belly. We breathed in the softness of skin, accentuated by our rough jeans.

"Your breasts are perfect." She held them cupped in her hands.

"I like yours." I circled her nipples with the palms of my hands. Nancy's were smaller and rounder than mine, with pale, almost white fuzz between them.

My fingers moved down to her waist and undid the buttons on her jeans. I held her hips against me, pressed her pelvis to mine. Kneeling slowly, I slid her pants over her legs, kissed her thighs, knees, calves. She sat on the bed to kick off her shoes; removed jeans and socks with one quick movement.

I stood in front of her, looked down on her cradled between my legs. Lifting her head to meet my gaze, she unzipped my pants in silence, kissed my belly. I leaned into her, arching my back. Her fingers traced circles around my protruding pelvis. The surrounding silence was broken only by our shallow breaths.

Hands on shoulders, I pushed her gently back onto the bed. Nancy raised her eyebrows, questioning, and laughed nervously. Lying beside her, I stroked her cheek, her brows, caressing and comforting, until her eyes closed, features smoothed. The flickering lamplight played on our features, danced over our heads. I drew her to me, kissed her cheeks, nose, ears, until our mouths met. Gently, then with increased passion, we held each other and rocked. The hum of passion turned to groans, turned to a roaring deep inside me.

Full, complete in our knowledge and ourselves, we began the ancient celebration. I moved on top of her, brushing her lips with a light kiss. My knee nestled between her legs, I crouched above her. A whimper escaped Nancy when my lips found her nipple, sucked nourishment, sucked fire, sucked life's energy.

My hands explored the curves of her body, the smoothness of tight skin over ribs. I stroked the softness of her belly, each caress a whirlpool, each revolution firmer, lower, deeper; her moans turned to a thin gasp as my fingers first brushed, circled, then gently held her pubes. I lay, still as a doe at the forest's edge, prolonging the first finger touch. My head on her breast, she cradled me with her legs. Her blood's heat, our matching pulse, moved my fingers and the rhythm quickened.

My mouth, no longer content with kisses, sought the lips of her other mouth. Her limbs seemed weightless as, head thrust back, back arched, she welcomed me. I gently touched her vulva, quivering, moist; slowly I fell into her folds. My tongue slid through her smooth passageway and outlined the mound of her clitoris, rising and pulsing in passion. My fingertips stroked the down of her lower back.

Again we paused, but not to rest; we had come too far for fatigue to catch us. Our hearts pounding, she looked at me wildly for a moment, disbelieving. I reached into her womb and heat flooded out as she opened to receive me. My tongue was its own agent now; it flickered, probed, dwelt, licked, sucked her juices until the screams echoed through her, through me, through the universe of our bodies, glistening with sweet sweat. We listened, spellbound, as the waves of pleasure washed through us.

Whispering my love, I moved up to feel the pressure of her body. Nancy lay motionless and tried to steady her breathing. Still shaking slightly, we held each other, fitting our curves together. She pulled my hair gently, gathering it in her fists. Our bodies stretched to their supple limit as all sensation was focused on those parts of us touching. My nipples rose in expectation as she pressed her mouth to my breasts. She sucked forcibly like a newborn who knows what she wants and how to get it. I wished all the milk I'd never held into her waiting mouth, so hungry for my pleasure.

Her hands followed the outline of my curves; we lay beside one another and explored the subtle differences of our bodies by touch, sight, smell. Her hands on my body created all the women I'd ever known, ever hoped someday I would be. All blended to her touch. My heart expanded to contain the joy of our being together and our powerful pleasure.

Nancy turned around and lay beside me, gently spreading my legs. My body cried for contact, but I did not want to force her with my desire. Slowly her fingers adventured, stroking, then opening the velvet folds. I wrapped my arms around her thighs and writhed as wisps of smoke, then fire ached through me.

Wet and open to her, I reached for her nerve. Nancy shook her head slightly and frowned, as if concentrating on my pleasure. She rubbed my moist lips, stroking my clitoris with increased tempo. I shuddered, moving under her.

I needed nothing now but Nancy inside me. She knew, moved to enter me but stopped suddenly, as if surprised by some unfamiliar landscape. Quivering with anticipation, my legs pulled inward and up. Sure of the power of my abandonment, I pressed my pelvis against her arm. She reached into me, pushed deeper and deeper until she was fast against the wall. My body hollowed with the tides of orgasm, I felt her fingers throughout me. I shouted my ecstasy into the night, scattering ripples of white light, shimmering heat of our passion.

The hum that was a roar was now a buzz in our inner ears, first to awaken from our daze. The moon had long since vanished; carefully we rearranged ourselves to suit the bed's form, pulled the covers up to our necks. She opened her mouth to speak; seemed to change her mind, was silent.

"Shhhhh," I whispered. "It's okay." I put my arm under her head; she turned into me, her arm hugging my side, her knees curled under her. I kissed her forehead lightly. She smiled, already asleep.

I woke the next morning to the sun streaming through the window, reflecting the glow I felt inside. Nancy still curled around me, her long hair trailing the pillow. Filled with an energy that overflowed my normal morning reflections, I stretched and gently disentangled our still moist bodies. Nancy groaned softly, pulling the quilt over her head.

"Morning, sunshine." I kissed the top of her head, the only part of her visible. No answer, so I ducked my head under the covers and, with my belly curled into her hip, laid my head on her breast and sucked her nipple, rising rapidly in anticipation.

"What are you doing now?" she asked, coming awake swiftly.

"My favorite position," I answered, massaging the underside slope of her breasts, down her rib cage to the curls of hair, then back to the waiting nipple. And it is; I have given up answering the male theorists who argue that it is my mother I secretly desire and the nourishment milk, not sexual satisfaction. I want it all, I decided: mother, milk, sex and a stiff nipple all mixed to fulfillment.

"My first orgasm last night was when you sucked my nipples," I said huskily with sleep and desire. "The next was when..."

And I laughed, sliding my hands along her smooth body, relishing her softness, our softness. I turned her gently onto her back and poised over her. Propped on my elbows, I looked into her face and smiled. I slid one arm around her neck, laid my head on her shoulder, kissed the nape of her neck lightly.

"Jackie, uh, not right now, okay? I want to wake up first, and—"

"Me too, usually. I mean, I like to be awake enough to enjoy it. I could help you open those baby blues of yours, though, if you want."

"What I want is to pee, and then I want tea and some of your bread with, let's see, rhubarb jam. Got any left?"

"Getting uppity, eh? I get the hint. Be right back."

Jumping up, I threw on a robe, slipped on a pair of moccasins and blew her a kiss from the door. Downstairs I worked swiftly, with none of my usual morning grogginess. The stove's fire blazed on the first match and I smiled approvingly. I got out the honey and cream, deciding to dust off the creamer that sat on the sill for ornament as a formal touch. I rearranged the flowers Nancy had given me yesterday for the tray. I hummed as I worked but what I wanted to do was shout, a big rebel yell of joy. The joy of rebels, a rebel of revelry; words joined and floated through my head while I finished making breakfast.

The tray was ready and I was just pouring the last of the water into the teapot when I heard Nancy's shoes on the stairs.

"Back in bed! You're about to get the grand treatment," I shouted when, turning, I saw her leaning, fully dressed, against the door.

"I gotta go." She sounded half sullen, half apologetic.

"Why? The animals can wait," I said slowly, trying not to anticipate disappointment.

"I'll call you soon."

"Call me?! You're just going to truck out the door and say you'll call me? You're crazy. If there's something on your mind, at least let me know. Nan?"

"You look so happy this morning. So complete. I'm scared."

I took in her words and her voice, forced myself to relax the knot in my throat.

"Oh, dear," I sighed. "Here, the tea's ready. Come on, sit down."

We sat in the same position as the evening before, and we both looked out the window at the dew on the grass, the pine tree near the garden, the beginnings of one of those special, warm, fall days. My initial panic left me, replaced by a new resolve.

"Nancy, what we did was good, it was right." My voice sounded too loud and forceful. "Was I too rough?" Softer this time, but I would not plead.

"No," both sad and braced for further admissions. She forced a tight smile. The sweet electricity of last night was now a charge between us.

"I know what you're thinking," I said, my mind racing and numb. "You're thinking our lives consist of a small town, neighbors we depend on and who depend on us. You're thinking it won't work. But there's nothing to 'work.' It happened."

"So?"

"So? What can I say? I can tell you I love you. I do. I'm a hopeless romantic, remember?"

"It's not just that, Jackie. It's other things, too."

"I know."

"Do you? I like my place in this community. You've got the

honor of being the town's eccentric. You even like it. You're so strong you don't need anyone else."

"I don't feel very strong right now." But I did, while my heart stretched to contain the hurt, a power was rising in me.

"Nancy," I continued, willing her to look at me. "You have given me so much support, so much strength. You've taught me how caring women can be, how loving. I've always hoped I give you the same."

"Last night was wonderful," Nancy replied. Whether she had heard what I was saying or not I couldn't tell. "I felt transported to the stars." She moved quickly to the other window, braced her back against the sink. "But I don't want to live in a space vacuum; I like it here at home, with Frank and the animals and discussing the price of flour over tea with my girlfriends." She frowned at the word, then looked me in the eyes clearly. "Of course I give you support. I relive your adventures and make them, in some ways, my own. That won't change. But neither will I. I don't want to."

"I don't want you to, either." I stared out the window, hypnotized by the sun. Finally I shrugged, got up to clear away the cups of now cold tea. I realized I wanted to move to the sink, to Nancy. I stood in the middle of the kitchen, feeling tired.

"Now you look sad. C'mon, wonderwoman, this will work out."

"It will, yes. But right now I think I'd like to be alone for a while."

"Okay," she said quickly, with a mixture of rejection and relief. "I'll call you soon. Or . . . come to supper tomorrow?"

"No, not tomorrow, but soon, I promise."

"I love you, Jackie."

"I'm glad. We'll see each other soon, really."

"All right." A hesitation, a quick shoulder hug, then Nancy

closed the door softly behind her.

I busied myself tidying a clean kitchen; paused only once, hearing Nancy's car turn down the gravel driveway. I wandered through the house, healing myself with its familiar sights and smells. Slowly, against all expectation, I found myself smiling.

"Oh, Nancy." Her name floated on the morning air; I pushed it with a kiss to the vanishing automobile, now climbing the rise. I love you, too, I thought. More and more. Not any more for last night; not any less for this morning. I looked in the dining room mirror, chuckling wryly, loving the hurt and the strength that even now sent tremors between my legs. Whew, girl, are you still horny? I thought, laughing and grimacing. Horny? You mean you haven't come up with a new name for this damp trembling yet, O woman of many words? Wombish? God, no. Yonish?

I slid my boots on over a pair of wool socks. Not bothering to dress, I slipped outside, the ties of my robe dragging through the wet grass. Hugging my breasts against the gooseflesh rising on my skin, I let the sun soak through the morning chill of land and body. Inhaling the morning air, I surveyed the last of the garden and the distant, gray bay. Yawning, I stretched my arms heavenward. Giving thanks, I moved out to greet the day.

# III

# THE FORBIDDEN

The dirty, the naughty and the forbidden have always been aspects of sexuality that for many people heighten the sexual experience. This attraction to the forbidden may date back to adolescence, when sexuality is shrouded in mystery, where the camouflage and innuendo make it all that much more desirable. Years later, even when sex has become quite acceptable, sexual acts that remain connected to the prohibited may continue to be highly arousing. And aspects of the illicit often become major themes in a person's fantasy life. Fantasies of making love with the possibility of being caught, with a stranger, with another couple or with a group of people are among the most common fantasies involving the forbidden.

Some people preserve their fantasies by refusing to risk enacting them in real life. They feel that reality can never be as good as fantasy and attempting to act out a fantasy would only ruin it. However, others pursue the forbidden fantasy and seize the opportunity when it presents itself. When an illicit real-life experience meets or surpasses a fantasy, it assumes tremendous stature, a unique moment stolen from an otherwise routine existence. Over a third of the stories in this volume are based on incidents which were unique or unusual. And because of this quality they were highly erotic experiences for the women involved.

### Group Sex

Possibly the single most popular sexual fantasy is one that includes sex with more than one partner. Most people never have the opportunity to try out this fantasy in real life, and continue to enjoy the experience in their mind's eye. Among those who do, many are disappointed. The potential for physical awkwardness, discomfort and jealousy can turn the experience into more of a nightmare than a dream. However, for Tashery Shannon, author of "Morning Light," a long-held fantasy was even better in reality. "I always had the fantasy of having sex with two men," said Tashery. "So I let the older brother know that I wanted to do that. When I met the younger brother and he was equally attractive to me, it seemed like a good idea. The actual experience was different from, but as good as or even better than, the fantasy. It had none of the bad undertones that could have been present with two brothers. I've had a few experiences of threesomes and foursomes since that time, and I have become aware of what it takes to make it work. It can be good as long as no one is threatened. If one person falls in love with one of the others or if someone else comes into the picture it can wreck it. It takes special people who are not possessive. These brothers were very close. They would call each other 'brother' and would share their most private thoughts. In fact, I was not the first woman they had shared; they had dated other women at the same time. But this was the first time they had ever made love together with the same woman. And it worked out well for them, too."

A sense of the illicit was what Helen Thomas found so exciting about making love with another couple in "California Quartet." "It was like entering a forbidden garden," she said. "There was joy in the naughtiness and knowing my friends would die or my mother would throw me in the cellar if they knew. Part of the thrill came from doing it and knowing that nice girls don't do such things." But the forbidden alone would not have been sufficient for Helen. The high caliber of the men involved was essential to her willingness to depart from her usual conservative patterns and abandon herself to a whole new experience. Says Helen, "This experience added a new dimension to sex because I'm usually a very private, conservative and traditional person, but the two men were so high powered and the house was so gorgeous that a whole mood was created. I didn't want to ruin the mood by walking away, and even though this kind of group experience was never a fantasy of mine, walking away from it would have left me feeling really disappointed. It was great for my ego because I played a pivotal role. By going with the flow, I cemented the experience."

Not only was the experience fun but Helen felt it added a dimension of depth to her relationship with her partner. "You can't plan or preordain such an experience," Helen said. "It's a trick of fate, but by participating I experienced a breakthrough in my own development. Part of bonding and growing together is sharing unusual experiences, and neither of us had ever done anything like this before. It made us closer and made me feel more attracted to him because he was generally very conservative, and I was seeing another side of him."

For the author of "Rub-a-Dub-Dub..." the experience of making love simultaneously to two men bypassed the normal concerns and awkwardness that accompany sex with a person for the first time and resulted in a deep, enduring friendship between the three of them. "Because two men were involved, there were none of the usual pressures to force the relationship into a more committed mold just because it was sexual," she said. "As a result, we were free just to love each other as friends." The author adds, "The fact that more than two people were involved also increased the possibilities for eroticism and variety. And since the two partners were men, I was the center of attention, which was just fantastic. It was so far beyond the

ordinary that it couldn't be programmed; it was totally spontaneous. And in this case, since we were all so comfortable
with each other, the whole evening was especially warm and
loving."

All of the senses are more highly stimulated when another
person or couple is involved in the sexual experience. Even
when the people involved are not physically touching each
other, the stimulation of watching or being watched, listening
or being overheard while in the throes of lovemaking can
intensify the whole experience. Overhearing the sounds of
lovemaking in the next room was incredibly erotic to the author
of "Evesdropping." But it was the mental images she could
generate, having never met her roommate's partner, that added
an additional turn-on. "The sounds were so erotic that it became voyeuristic," she said. "And the fact that I had never met
the man and didn't even know what he looked like allowed
incredible room for fantasy during the experience and made it
even more erotic."

### Anonymous Sex

If an unknown partner in the next room can provide material
for fantasy, interacting with a partner who is a perfect stranger
allows the imagination absolute free reign. Both people can
assume any personas they desire. With no image to uphold
and no relationship to be concerned about, some people find
it easier to abandon themselves more completely to the physical sexual experience. The lack of inhibition created by anonymous sex can intensify both the sexual experience and their
enjoyment of it.

For Susan Block, not knowing her partner allowed her not
only to build a fantasy around him, but to superimpose dream-

like fantasy images over the entire event. According to Susan, "The experience in 'Women Who Love Men Who Love Horses' captured the part of me that enjoys fantasy. It happened so quickly that it was like a dream; so I could include the dreamlike images of the horses. Since I didn't know this guy very well, I could project a fantasy onto him. I could make him into whatever I wanted him to be."

For the author of "The Moon Over SoHo" it was the aspect of being able to assume a fantasy role herself that was both protective and enticing. "The zipless fuck is a fantasy world that I can enter. It's a game," she said. "I can use a false name and false details about my life like saying I'm younger or older. This way I'm anonymous so they can't know the real me. Not having this self-consciousness enables me to feel more sexual." The author continues on a more personal and revealing note, "Also, I have this self-dislike that goes way back and I think that if someone knew me, they wouldn't like me. Generally, I don't think of myself as sexy. I'm treated by most people as an intellectual. But as a pure female object in a brief encounter, I can feel really sexy."

Because of the real possibility of danger, most people think of men and not women seeking anonymous sex. Most men are stronger physically and, with good reason, many women hesitate to expose themselves to the dangers involved in being so physically vulnerable. However, the writers who wrote about anonymous sexual experiences said that, at the time, they were not conscious of the dangers. As one author said, "When I was younger, I would pick men up. I had a willful innocence and I never considered a man would be dangerous. I never considered for a minute that I'd be hurt. Although, now that I look back on it, I feel I was very lucky." Another noted, "I feel nostalgia for those days when doing stuff like that was possible.

I felt just like a guy going out to score. I've outgrown that phase now, and concerns about health would prevent me from doing it anyway, but I loved it when it was happening, and I never felt afraid."

In general, the "zipless fuck" is totally unanticipated. An opportunity avails itself and is seized, almost before conscious evaluation can take place. Carol Conn, in "A Very Special Dance," was primed for such an encounter by the sultry environment of a local reggae club. According to Carol, "The reggae music, the people there, as a matter of fact, the atmosphere of the entire club was charged with a sexual rhythmic energy. The whole environment was sexual and sensual. All of this made way for the unknown person to be accepted, even desired, in this unusual situation."

And it's the unusual situation, the illicit, the forbidden, that stuff of which fantasies are made, that can create real yet unique sexual experiences, as shown by the following stories.

# GROUP SEX

## *Morning Light*

### BETH TASHERY SHANNON

When Brian left Kentucky for a month, it couldn't have been more natural than for his brother Stephen and me to talk about certain things.

Carrying the horses their feed in the morning, I began, "I wish Brian wouldn't shut me out whenever he feels bad."

Later, shoveling muck, Stephen muttered, "My brother thinks that just because he's older he's always right."

"I'm glad he cares about people, but he thinks he's got to keep the whole world from crashing down," I called that afternoon as I cleaned the feet of the horse I'd just brought in.

"And doesn't notice it can hold itself up just fine," Stephen answered from the next stall.

As we trotted the two Arabians along the shoulder of the hill to the rolling open spaces where we could gallop, I found myself getting around to it. "Sometimes he could do better at not taking me for granted in bed, too."

Hours later, Stephen answered, "Everybody gets taken for granted. I wish people could stop seeing me as Brian's little brother, and see *me*."

I looked down from the bench where I was sitting to Stephen on the barn floor, his back propped against baled flakes of alfalfa, his arms around his knees. Sunlight angling through a high window lit his hair to a gold much paler than Brian's, and

fell across the slender arms that were tanned the color of a
lion's hide. He was frowning, his head down so his eyes were
almost hidden by the curls of his hair. His straight nose and
small mouth were much more finely made than his brother's.

And here I was, guilty of just what he'd been talking about.
Brian and Stephen stuck close as two burrs, running the board-
ing stable together, fixing up the place together. For the first
time it occurred to me that after six months with Brian, I didn't
even know what Stephen did when he wasn't working the
horses or shoveling out his share of the stalls.

He glanced up at me, and in the slanting light his eyes
glowed startling blue above his high, narrow cheekbones—
the blue you see in pictures of exotic butterflies.

What happened that night seemed perfectly natural, too.
I'd thought of Stephen as a kid, when in some ways he was
every bit as mature as Brian. Still, that young eagerness to
please was unspoiled in Stephen; the riding muscles in his long
thighs and narrow back were slender and graceful, and he
wanted me not once or twice that night, but many times.

During those four weeks we knew better than to talk about
what would happen when Brian got back to Kentucky. I was
making no plans to lie to Brian. If he really meant all we'd
agreed on about "love" not meaning "own," he'd just have to
accept it. But I was afraid he hadn't meant his brother when
we'd talked about other lovers. I couldn't see any way to avoid
making a choice between the two, and I dreaded it.

As it turned out, Brian got back too full of all he'd done in
San Francisco for me to jump in and mention anything right
away. Stephen and I listened to his stories sitting on the arena
fence side by side, but a little apart. If Brian noticed anything,
I couldn't tell.

And then Brian and I got off alone, and it was better than

I'd remembered just to watch the dark blond beauty of him, the browned skin sliding over the mature shapes of his muscles like water over rounded stones, and to feel the familiar sureness of his touch. Stroking open his full, slightly pouting lips with mine, I tasted the warm, responsive sweetness of his tongue while our hips moved slowly together, and every touch of him in me opened me to him again, down to my core. He answered me with openness.

I was ready to take my favorite mare out, the little chestnut Arabian, slightly pigeon-toed. I gave her a quick once-over and went for her saddle. As I pulled up the stool to reach her bridle off its high nail, Stephen walked into the tack room. "Come look at this."

"What?"

"Out here," he answered, then turned and headed out. It was plain that was all the answer I was going to get, so I left the bridle hanging and followed him out to the stalls. He headed for the empty one he'd been spreading with fresh straw for a new boarder who was supposed to show up in the after-noon. He stopped just inside the stall door.

"What? I don't see anything."

"You didn't look hard enough."

I turned around in the stall, gazing at the white painted walls, the window full of morning light and leafy shade, the stall floor thickly covered with new straw. From behind, Stephen's arm wrapped around my waist, and he nuzzled the back of my neck.

"Not now," I told him. "No telling who might walk in." Really, I wasn't sure if we should again, anytime.

"Brian's fixing the fence in the far pasture." His lips closed over my earlobe, and he sucked gently.

"One of the boarders might come."

"I shut the barn door. We'd hear way before anybody could get in." Stephen reached to the door of the stall and slid it closed too, then he turned to face me. With his high, angular cheeks and vivid blue eyes he looked translucent in the early light, and suddenly fragile.

I shook my head no, but he saw I wasn't sure. He moved closer, and I could smell the fragrance of straw and alfalfa on him as he pressed his slender thighs to mine through our jeans. Light as a fern, his tongue brushed my lower lip, and at the same time I felt him opening my top shirt button.

"We shouldn't do this, Stephen," I told him, hearing how weak my words sounded.

"Don't do nothing, then. Stay like that." He unbuttoned my shirt, pulled it off and unfastened my bra. His cool hands stroked my breasts, then he bent his head and moist, living warmth flowed around my nipples, sending little shivers up my spine. I leaned toward him, still shaking my head no, but laughing at the game it had become. I opened and pushed off his shirt too, and stroked his lean back down the little ridges of his backbone to the two indentations just above his pants and the swell of his buttocks. The hair there was a soft, fine fuzz. He didn't notice me stroking, he was too busy tugging my jeans down. I stepped out of them and lay in the straw, closing my eyes. Little ends of straw poked my back and the fresh smell of it rose around me, reminding me of other times with Stephen, and shaking all the resolve I'd made the night before to leave him alone.

I felt him pull down my underpants, and his hands closed lightly around my hips. Then he moved up and our tongues slid warm together. With my eyes shut, all I could see was a vaguely pulsing swirl of red that seemed the same as the movements of our mouths and the eager, gentle searching of his hand between my legs.

A rumbling started at the far end of the barn, and grew louder. I sat up. Stephen rocked back to a crouch, his nostrils flaring.

The door rumbled shut, and steps sounded in the barn. If it was only a boarder, their horses were mostly in the stalls at the far end, but even a boarder would have to go past us to the tack room, and the door of our stall had a barred window, with no way to close it. Our only chance of not being seen was to huddle silent where we were. As quietly as I could, I fumbled to untangle my underpants and get them on. Steps sounded in the aisle and came nearer.

The stall door rattled back.

Brian stood looking down at us. Stephen scrambled away from me as if he'd been shocked by electricity. I managed to untwist my underpants, but it was too late. There I lay naked, legs spread in the straw.

"Caught you both!" For a second I thought his voice was uneven with anger, then I heard the laughter just beneath. His eyes met mine only briefly, like a dare. Once I'd made a joking threat to him that someday I'd grab both him and his brother and fuck them together. He'd laughed and told me to go ahead.

Brian frowned fiercely at Stephen. "Quit scooting around, brother! Too late to get dressed now." He glanced at me again, and this time it was definite—the laughter and the dare. "Think I'm dumb, huh?" he asked us. Then with one quick movement he pulled his shirt over his head and threw it down, dusty from horses and work. A fine film of dust covered the smooth brown skin of his chest. I stared at him. The day I'd threatened to grab him and Stephen, he'd known that under my teasing I really wanted to. But I had never thought he meant what he had said, too.

Brian unzipped his jeans, let them drop, pulled them off with his boots and stood, hand on his hip, while Stephen in his corner gawked, astonished.

The soft light made the ripples and hollows of Brian's body seem to glow. His cock wasn't erect, but it had that full, heavy look. "I can share, if you can," he told Stephen.

Stephen glanced at me, as if for help.

"Well, brother?" Brian asked.

Then I saw how Brian was watching me too, baiting me on purpose by pretending the decision had nothing to do with me.

"Maybe I don't want to," I answered him, playing at dignity. If you can be dignified lying jaybird-naked on a stall floor.

Before I could say more, Brian knelt over me, holding down my hands. "I'll keep her down while you eat her, then let's trade!"

In his corner Stephen was smiling now, obviously relieved that Brian was playing instead of really being angry at him.

"Get fucked," I told Brian, and pretended to kick him, but I was laughing too hard, both at Brian's game and at the effect it was having on his brother.

When Stephen saw it was all right with me, he pushed off his jeans and boots with a great show of casualness and tossed them backward into a corner. Then he sat closer to us, uncertain what to do or say next.

"Dare you," I challenged them both.

Without letting my wrists loose, Brian leaned down and covered my mouth with his, pushing his tongue in. I bit it, but gently, while peeking at Stephen.

Stephen gave his brother a quick glance, but he too was grinning. Finally, he leaned over to give me a kiss. Brian moved back and made room for Stephen, then Stephen made way for Brian again. Alternating back and forth was fun, but it was still more playful than passionate, and I was starting to hope for something more. I slipped my hands out of Brian's loose grasp and pulled both men close, Brian's muscular smoothness on one of my breasts, Stephen's slender, gold-fuzzed chest on the other. I smiled up at them and stroked their hair, Stephen's bright, curly and fine, Brian's darker and longer, in loose waves. All four of their hands caressed me at once.

Part of me wanted to wonder about it, whether this was supposed to be a play at sex that meant nothing, or a whole new arrangement between the three of us that could open up a complicated can of worms. But the worms were already out of the can, and even as I started to worry, I found myself closing my eyes and sinking into the pure contentment of being stroked by both of them. For a while I tried to guess who was where, but I couldn't. They moved from one nipple to the other, sometimes sucking one at a time, sometimes both together. One minute I'd feel Brian's tongue swirling around and around, then a second later on the same nipple, Stephen's hungry sucking while Brian's tongue flicked rapidly over my other nipple. Sometimes I suspected them of leaning toward each other's side, trying to fool me, till finally I completely lost track, like one floating anchorless on a warm ocean, out of sight of land.

A hand stroked my thighs, and I parted my legs to whoever it might be. A tongue slid wet over my cunt, down between the sensitive folds of skin, then lapped at my inner lips. At the same time another tongue centered on my clit, startling me.

As I looked down, there were two heads, pale gold and deep gold, crowded close, moving slightly with their licking. Like two ponies sharing a salt block, I couldn't help thinking, but I kept from laughing. Each made way for the other, nuzzling together till pale and tawny, curly and wavy hair blended together. I loved the ease of their bodies resting so intimately, belly brushing hip, thigh grazing thigh, though they would probably have been shocked if I'd mentioned any such thing. Stephen's honey-colored hips and buttocks were narrow, his cock half hard and tapering at the head like a delicate sculpture, and Brian's body was somehow both more coarse and yet more finely made, his cock curving upward, its head large, well defined, yet peculiarly graceful like the rest of him. The pink of Brian's nipples and the dark gold of the hair above his cock were the same as Stephen's. Both brothers were lapping with one rhythm now, tongues flicking over me from the left, then from the right. I touched their heads again, one with each hand, urging them to come forward to my clit.

They did, sometimes tongues together, sometimes one ever so slightly behind the other, making a quick double rhythm that caught me unawares. Little flares of greedy arousal sparked through me. I twisted my hips in their hands and clutched fistfuls of straw, raising myself eagerly to their mouths.

Simultaneously they lifted their heads, glanced at each other and grinned. Then they lowered their heads to me again, cheeks pressed together, renewing their double-time rhythm. Flickerings of warmth crept up my spine and down my thighs. With my eyes shut and my head thrown back I felt the stroking and kneading of Stephen's narrow, long fingers and Brian's broad, sensitive hands over my whole body, their tongues waking a heat that radiated from my cunt till the flickerings became one long, urgent need and bright, shuddering waves broke through. I cried out and sank my fingers hard into their backs, not caring who heard me, aware only of their arms around me, their bodies pressing hard and yet yielding to mine.

A loud, impatient thump sounded behind my head. I jerked up, away from it. Thump, bump! Then a quiet snuffling. The chestnut mare next door. "She says turn down the noise," Stephen said, laughing. I settled back against the wall while

Stephen stroked my stomach, playing with his thumb around my navel.

I held out my arms to him, and as he eased into them, he continued to kiss me. For a while we snuggled and rubbed together while Brian sat with his back against the wall, close by but not touching us. Stephen's kisses grew more intense but felt more desperate than passionate. "What's the matter?" I finally whispered.

For an answer, he pressed his cock to me. It had become soft and small. "Did you tell him about us?" he asked me abruptly.

I shook my head no.

"I knew you'd end up together," Brian said.

"What, this morning?"

"No," Brian answered, stretching his legs out easily in the straw. "I thought so even before I left."

Stephen made an exasperated movement. "Then why didn't you say anything?"

"What, give you permission? It was no business of mine."

"Well," Stephen answered, "I don't mind sharing, but I won't go first."

I traced the curve of Stephen's back. "Feel like watching?"

"Sure," he said with relief and moved quickly aside.

Brian shook his head, pretending to be shocked, but stretched out beside me. He opened my lips with his and sucked my bottom lip gently. I put my arms around him, feeling the strong warmth of him along the whole length of me. He thrust his hips slowly forward, and I closed my fingers over the shaft of his cock and stroked it in a lazy rhythm.

Stephen sat under the window, watching us with open curiosity. I moved down to Brian's balls, and still rubbing his cock, licked and sucked the kidskin softness of them, partly to arouse Brian, and partly to arouse Stephen.

"How does it feel, brother?" Stephen asked after a while, but whether he was playing along out of nervousness or really turned on, I couldn't tell.

"Pretty good," Brian answered in a tone that was meant to be casual but had a soft edge to it like the sound of a cat talking and purring at the same time.

I licked up the shaft of his cock to the head and took it into my mouth, dwelling on all his favorite places, around the ridge, up the underside of the head. Closing my eyes I took him completely into my mouth in long, rolling sucks till the bland-salt drops welled from him. He pulled me down beside him and faced me, positioning his swollen, moist cock to my opening.

Stephen was leaning forward, elbows in the straw, watching us. Brian felt me looking at him. Glancing over his shoulder with one eye cracked open he said, "Excuse us a minute, brother, while we get incoherent." Then he slid his hips toward me and pressed in.

I guided his cock as it slipped easily into the wet of my cunt. Just the feel of him so hard, warm and alive, so definitely present at the center of me, sent swift fountains of delight through me. I wrapped my legs over his round, tight ass, easing him farther in, and we began a leisurely movement together, lingering over each sensation. From where Stephen sat I knew he could see our joining as Brian's cock disappeared and reappeared between my wet, swollen inner lips. I wondered if it seemed ugly to him, or sexy, or maybe beautiful. Knowing he was there but not being able to see him made me feel self-conscious and yet turned on in a way I'd never felt before. It gave me a feeling of being doubly vulnerable that almost scared me. But Brian lay equally unguarded with his head pillowed on my arm. The veins of his neck were large from his deliberately slow movements. The uncompromising, unselfconscious beauty of him quieted my uneasiness. I kissed him again and rolled onto him. He thrust his hips up to meet me, entering so deep I felt pierced, while a pang of intense delight curled and uncurled still deeper within me. We pushed toward each other, craving some further meeting, in short, frantic motions, and our lips fastened hard together as flame shot between us, creating a streaming, molten river that dissolved the walls of our skin and veins, washing us past the sunlight-striped stall, beyond everything as our blood melted into a single, bright liquid flame.

Slowly we turned over, and Brian sighed, letting his head fall onto my shoulder. I stroked the dampness between his shoulder blades, floating in a vague, blissful haze of the smell of straw mingled with sex.

I heard a rustling close to my ear, as Brian was pushed to the side. Grinning, but without bothering to open his eyes, he rolled off me, and I couldn't help but grin, too, as I put my arms around Stephen. "Impatient, huh?" I teased him in a whisper.

But in spite of his bravado his smile was still a little embarrassed. I kissed him, taking a long while as I cradled the long slenderness of his cock in my hand. Stephen's cock hair was the softest I'd ever touched. "You're my dessert," I whispered in his ear, "the sweetest part."

But he raised his head, frowning at me. "Is that all?"

I met the questioning blue of his eyes, and saw the playful challenge ready to cover hurt. In the last month I'd come to really see that expression of his for the first time.

"No," I answered. "No, that's not nearly all. You're somebody I love." I kissed him, and he responded eagerly. Still he was playful, but this time his play held no hidden hurt. He rubbed his hips and belly on mine and began to enter me. I tilted my hips so he could sink in deeply. He glanced toward his brother, but Brian smiled at him and shut his eyes. Stephen smiled at Brian, and at me, and began the tumblebugging he liked so much, one of us on top, then the other, rolling in the straw till we raised a fine gold dust and little pieces of straw clung all over our damp skin. Each time we slid together it was at a different angle and with a whole different sensation. Echoes of my coming reverberated in me, and I held Stephen close, our hearts beating together, our tongues meeting and licking more like foals' than people's. His eagerness woke an answering tenderness in me, and I felt myself open yet more deeply to him. His hunger made me hungry, and I shivered with the kind of desire that builds after not making love for weeks. My whole womb felt as if it was swirling and shuddering around him. "Does it feel good?" he panted, anxious even in his passion.

I nodded yes, struggling to keep from hollering with its goodness and spooking every horse in the barn. He collapsed on me, plunging his hips as spasms shot up through me like some rare flower bursting open and slowly, gradually, dissolving away.

Dimly, in the recesses of my awareness, I felt a familiar warmth beside me. A strong arm pillowed my head, and another stroked my side. I turned my face to Brian and our lips and tongues flowed lazily together. Then Stephen's smaller, clear-cut lips brushed mine, as languid as water subsiding after a flood.

It all felt more natural and comfortable than I could ever have dared to hope. Nearly perfect. Only one final action remained. I opened my eyes and looked at both of them. "Come here, you two," I said as I raised my lips to theirs. And our three mouths met in a long, leisurely kiss as we rested the warmth of our bodies tenderly together.

# California Quartet

## HELEN A. THOMAS

"Darling," he said, running his thumb absentmindedly over the top of my hand, "I hope my cousin has provided chilled wine for us."

Taking Kurt's fingers and kissing them one by one, I murmured, "Surely Arthur would not offer his hospitality for the evening without the amenities. Of course there will be wine." Even though Kurt and Arthur had not seen each other in years, Arthur would have to realize that his international businessman relative, head of a Canadian conglomerate, suffered only the best of anything. Poor wine or no wine at all would be a serious omission in entertaining someone like Kurt.

Before closing the glass shield that separated us from the chauffeur, Kurt handed him the address. The location was unfamiliar to me—an obscure road off the San Diego Freeway. Picturing a small cottage or an ageing California ranch house, I was surprised when the long white limousine pulled up in front of an exclusive cluster of condominiums with tall iron gates and a security guard. Multistory houses with red tile roofs, surrounded by lush landscaping, were in stark counterpoint to the dull dryness of the mountaintop. The limo slithered through the gates to Arthur's house, which appeared wider and taller than the others.

"What does Arthur do?" I asked Kurt.

"Writes for television," he answered.

"He must write a lot," I murmured.

"Whatever he does," Kurt said, appraising the situation, "he does it well."

An Oriental houseman in a white jacket appeared at the car door. He bowed ever so slightly, almost imperceptibly, and announced, as we had already known, that Arthur would be late. He guided us to a guest room off the foyer, where we could change into our bathing suits.

"Let's look at the house first," Kurt suggested, taking me by the elbow. Hand in hand we wandered through Arthur's min-icastle. A sweeping staircase curved downward from the second floor. A white grand piano rested in the alcove formed by the curved bannister. The living room was all in white. Thick white rugs. White walls. White velvet love seats, pristine and spar-kling. A huge black urn, glazed and shiny, held immense black silk orchids on a low white table. White silk shades crowned acrylic lamps.

"My cousin does have a flair for the dramatic," Kurt com-mented.

The upstairs rooms were more normal, decorated in a variety of colors and prints, with beds unmade, couches rumpled, and the bathroom floor strewn with towels. In the study—large, sunny, and airy—Kurt and I ran our eyes over the leather-bound books of Arthur's television scripts. A group of Oriental erotic prints were arranged over the massive desk. Kurt smiled at the sight of the figures engaged in anal sex beneath volu-minous kimonos. Responding to the art, he slid his hand up my skirt and squeezed my buttocks playfully. I squeezed his in return. He allowed a finger to stray between my legs, unen-cumbered by underthings, and commented on the moist re-ception. "Is it the company or the art, darling?" he asked as he took me into his arms, kissing me and fondling me with quick, strong fingers.

"You're going to arouse me," I said, laughing and pulling away.

"That is a *fait accompli,* my dear," he said, producing a wet finger as evidence. "Methinks the lady is ready already."

"It's you, Kurt," I said, gazing at him fondly. "Let's swim. Love is for later." I kneaded the front of his khaki trousers, feeling warmth exude through the fine silk fabric. Just a little teasing and taunting, I thought, staring into his sapphire eyes, inscrutable in boardrooms but transparent to me.

Kurt is tall and fair. He looks as Nordic and Germanic as his name. His beard, trimmed to the contours of his face, is blond—flecked with gray, as is his hair. At sixty, he is conscious of his age, but he is vital, lusty, seductive and attentive. And sexy.

He followed me downstairs where we undressed. I noted his semierection and bent down to run my tongue tauntingly over it, enjoying the stiffening response. We both knew that after we swam, we would return to this room and make leisurely love. But we had both underestimated our host.

Arthur's backyard met even Kurt's jet-set standards. A long elegant pool dominated the space. Blue-green water shimmered in the last light of late afternoon. Masses of semitropical shrubs bordered the enclosed area, which smelled vaguely of honeysuckle. Persian cats scampered in the back, and a pair of brightly colored parrotlike birds watched us from their exotic cage built into the side of a rock.

"My cousin does not lack for imagination," Kurt stated dryly.

"All we need is peacocks meandering about," I said.

"Into the water, Maria," he ordered, diving in. We swam seriously for some time. Kurt's long, lean body—muscled and hard—glided through the water gracefully. My strokes were slower but equally rhythmical. When I felt exhausted by the exercise, I climbed out of the pool and removed my cap, allowing my damp auburn hair to fall to my shoulders. Kurt followed me, slapping me on my bottom.

"This calls for a drink," he said, towel-drying himself.

Accustomed to the dwindling light and the onslaught of darkness, we were both astonished when paper lanterns, heretofore unnoticed, were suddenly illuminated, lending a fairyland quality to the garden. Small white lights trailing over the treetops twinkled. Then, classical music—heavy with flutes and violins—flooded the air.

Startled, Kurt and I looked at each other and then laughed merrily at the theatrics of it all.

Swathed in large, white towels with gray monograms, we padded into the kitchen to find a silver ice bucket with Louis Cristal champagne and a tray of cheeses, breads, pâtés and grapes. The houseman appeared out of nowhere and announced *sotto voce*, "I will bring it to you."

"We are going to get out of our wet suits first," Kurt said.

In the little guest room we found white terry-cloth robes draped on the sofa. "Arthur thinks of everything," Kurt said. "I am impressed with my relative."

As we slipped out of our wet suits, Kurt drew me to him, naked and chilled from the water. "I want to feel your breasts against my chest," he said, kissing me behind the ear. We lingered with the kiss while my hand lovingly cupped his genitals, damp, limp and in need of encouragement. "Later," I whispered, my voice full of promise.

"Later," he whispered back.

We returned poolside, in the robes, to find the champagne and hors d'oeuvres on a small table. Music filled the background and the night air was sweet.

Kurt brought me a fluted glass of champagne. He sat down

next to me on the chaise and opened my robe so that my bosom sparkled in the moonlight. He dribbled the wine over each breast, and then bent to lick it off, his tongue flicking my nipples gently in the process. He sucked each breast long enough to stir longings of desire in my groin. Then he closed my robe and returned to his own chaise.

"You look beautiful," he said softly. "I never cease to marvel at your breasts. You have the breasts of a young girl."

A booming voice from the house interrupted our dialogue. "Hallo, Kurt," shouted our host.

"Arthur," my lover called in return.

We both stood up to greet him.

A youthful replica of Kurt strode forward, bare-chested, wearing only a white sarong tied at his waist. A mat of gleaming, fine hair covered his chest. Not as many lines as Kurt's etched the high-cheekboned planes of his handsome face. No beard or mustache. His hair fell rakishly over his forehead in a charming manner, highlighting the mischievous twinkle in his blue eyes. His companion, a small, dark-haired woman, was also bare-chested and wearing only a sarong.

"Meet Jasmine," Arthur said, "and you must be Maria."

"Yes," I answered, surprised at his robust nature, so different from Kurt's quiet reserve.

He and Kurt embraced. "How do you like California, old man?" Arthur asked.

"Ouch," Kurt said, wincing. "Old is right on target."

"Sorry," Arthur said, flicking off his sarong. "Have you been in the hot tub yet?"

"No," we answered simultaneously.

Arthur stood naked before us. Jasmine, pixieish—with no hips or tits—followed suit. I could not help staring at Arthur's penis—it looked like a rosebud nestled in a bed of fine flaxen hair. Jasmine's mound was as dark as Arthur's was light, and considerably more lush.

"This must be Hollywood," Kurt said with wry overtones.

"We planned a conservative, at-home evening for you," said Arthur, standing like a classical Greek statue, poised in front of the tub. "Is Kurt as prim and proper as ever?" he asked. "We haven't been together for years, you know. And he was always so well behaved."

"And you?" I asked, lifting my eyes that had been riveted to that spot between his legs.

"A little on the naughty side," he said, "always."

Then Arthur reached out for Jasmine's hand and led her into the tub.

"What now?" I asked Kurt.

"When in Rome," he said, shrugging his shoulders, allowing his robe to fall to the ground, exposing his nudity. He unfastened my robe and removed it from me. "I want them to see how beautiful you are," he whispered into my ear. This sudden interest in exhibitionism fascinated me. Kurt was ordinarily a very private person, cautious and offended at the slightest intrusion into his conservative habit patterns. Something about the evening was playing havoc with his libido and sensibilities. Taking my hand, he led me to the redwood deck. With uncertainty and some misgivings, I approached the tub, buoyed only by the glint in Kurt's eyes.

"What pretty breasts Maria has," crooned Jasmine, her voice crisp with a French accent.

Embarrassed, I muttered something unintelligible and was glad for the pressure of Kurt's protective hand on mine.

Kurt helped me into the tub. I almost tripped in the semi-darkness, and my celebrated left breast grazed Arthur's cheek. He reached up to touch it. I flinched and, in a moment, was seated between Kurt and Jasmine, with Arthur directly across from me.

Arthur called his houseman, who arrived in a flash with a tray of drinks. As the houseman moved away from us, toward the house, a colored light went on, spotlighting the tub. To my dismay, we could all see each other quite clearly, bathed in a diffused haze of colored illumination. This new theatrical device made me laugh. Arthur was simply incorrigible with his toys! Glancing at Kurt, I could translate the curve of his lips and the look in his eye. I knew that he, too, was relaxing and that he was resigned to enjoying his cousin's dramatic, erotic tableau.

The water reached the top of my rib cage, just under my breasts, so that they skirted the water, rather like lotus blossoms floating on lily pads. My eyes moved to Jasmine, who was chattering in French to Arthur. Her nonexistent tits reached the same level. We four sat in the sweet, semitropical evening air, politely conversing in a Daliesque scenario.

The scene must have been arousing to Arthur, for his small rosebud had blossomed into an immense erection that stood straight out like an underwater flagpole. Jasmine's hand flew to Arthur's erect penis, as if guided there by radar. She interjected comments in French into the conversation and quickly translated them into English, while fondling Arthur in a manner that was casual and offhand. Her impertinence fascinated me as much as our communal nudity.

A smile appeared on my face at the sight of Kurt's penis, also thrust forward, like a missile in search of a target. I was amused by his and my reaction to this supreme California hedonism. Kurt's toes touched mine, and I longed to reach over and touch his penis—long, hard, and inviting—but I sat there in puritanical psychic chains.

Jasmine knew no such restraints. She ducked underwater and took an all too delighted Arthur into her mouth, wrapping her tiny lips partway around his penis.

My eyes met Kurt's. We smiled at each other. I felt a tingling throughout my body.

Jasmine came up for air and then submerged once more.

"She won't suffer from a lack of oxygen, will she?" I asked.

"Not to worry, darling," Kurt offered, putting his hand between my legs. "I am sure Jasmine has the situation well in hand."

"Or well in mouth," I quipped, shivering with pleasure, enjoying the touch of Kurt's strong fingers pressing against tender places. I shifted to accommodate him, so that he could wiggle his fingers in and out.

Jasmine reappeared above water. Saying not a word but gargling with champagne, which she spewed out onto the grass, she turned to me playfully and repeated an earlier remark, "Maria has such pretty breasts."

A bit annoyed, I retorted, "You said that already."

Without further comment, she leaned over and put her mouth to my breast.

I was horrified. A feeling of repugnance overcame me. I was about to push her away when I felt Kurt's arm press down on mine—a command to remain still. Bemusement filled his eyes.

I glanced at Arthur.

He smiled.

My repulsion evaporated, superseded by a feeling of ecstasy.

Jasmine slid her tongue around, then without allowing her teeth to touch the surface of my skin, she suckled my breasts. The suckling created wave after wave of sensuous pleasure, heightened by her next move: she lifted her head ever so slightly and concentrated on just the nipple, biting the red, juicy hardness with darting nips. The staccato bites of her tiny, perfect white teeth caused a glorious tingling to pervade my being. Heat flooded down my spine. Her technique was flawless.

While her teeth still possessed me, she pushed Kurt's hand from between my legs and replaced it with her own finger, which moved in a rapidly increasing jabbing momentum, in and out, in and out.

The night seemed strange, unreal, remote. I felt disengaged from my body and completely helpless when a hand directed mine to Kurt's penis, which I grasped with fervor. I tried to match the pace set by Jasmine, stroking him with the same pulsating madness with which she stroked me. I had never been touched by a woman that way before. Were it not for Kurt, I would not have allowed it. Yet by now my objections were academic, as I thrilled to her flicking finger, her exploring tongue, her calculating mouth. Jasmine lifted her head from my breast. I wanted to shriek, "Don't stop," so exquisite were the sensations she created. Then I felt Kurt's familiar lips and mouth claim my other breast, the rough texture of his beard adding to the stunning tactile sensations and stimulating me even more. I stroked him with increased momentum, as he responded with a primitive passion. In contrast to the gentle, disciplined flicking and biting of Jasmine's trained lips, tongue and teeth, Kurt began gorging himself on me, taking all that his generous mouth could accommodate. Then he pulled back, licking my erect nipple with his lavish tongue. Time and space had retreated to the recesses of my mind. My senses reeled. I was aware of nothing but the pleasure, the sweetness of the night air and the clarity of the music in the background.

Kurt's desire flamed beyond his control. He brushed Jasmine aside and lifted me onto him. I felt the wondrous impact of his hardness as it penetrated my body. As I rode up and down on him, he pressed his mouth to mine, probing his ardent tongue between my lips. I was certain that he would come in an instant, but abruptly he pushed me off and jumped out of the water, his penis huge and formidable.

Kurt pulled me out after him and laid me down on the grass, damp from the touch of night. On bended knees he straddled me so that his penis fanned my face. Ribbons of moonlight darted across his body. Shadows danced in the backdrop. He seemed distant and, at the same time, so close that he was a part of me. I recognized my cue and took him hungrily into my mouth. The feel and taste of him excited me, as always. Spirals of delight spun through my being. With passion I sucked on his cock, feeding my growing appetite for him. Oblivious to everything but his moans, I lathered my tongue around his penis. He moved upward and downward, forward and backward, to increase his sensual pleasure.

I sensed someone watching. In the distance I noticed Arthur and Jasmine looking at us as they continued ministering to one another. They seemed to be transfixed, their eyes focused mindlessly on Kurt's massive cock sliding in and out of my mouth, in pursuit of my loving, relentless tongue. Their presence and attentiveness heightened my own experience. Shocked, I realized that I enjoyed their being there, as waves of heat swept through my lower body. All my reactions intensified. I wanted them to watch! I wanted to reach out and touch Arthur's penis. I wanted to touch Jasmine between her legs. Suddenly Kurt pulled away from my mouth, straightened his legs, and plunged his penis into me in a swift, almost vicious movement, as his swollen organ slid into my moist, anxious, awaiting vagina.

As Kurt thrust himself upward and forward, colliding with

the front wall of my vagina and hitting my cervix, spasms of excitement made me quiver. I moaned with pleasure. My sounds somehow made me aware that the others could hear. As I opened my eyes again I saw Jasmine and Arthur making love, as a new and exquisite sensation coursed through my body. I felt as if we were racing through space, spinning in a timeless chute, bypassing brilliant galactic lights, hurtling into the unknown.

Arthur stepped in back of Jasmine, wrapping one arm around her so that his fingers brushed her small nipples, his other arm extending toward her mound of hair. All the time Arthur's eyes were on us, as my eyes were on them. My own clitoris felt unusually sensitive and vulnerable as I watched Arthur fingering Jasmine.

Kurt's endurance bore testimony to the fact that he, too, derived some sensual, erotic drive from the onlookers. His grunts mounted with enthusiasm. He thrust himself in and out like a randy stallion, bringing me to heights that I had not experienced before. He pulled himself out, and in that one instant of seeing his cock shining in the moonlight, dripping with my love juices, I wanted Jasmine to suck on him. I wanted to watch. I wanted to suck Arthur. I wanted Arthur to suck me. I screamed, "Please, please, now," as Kurt plunged into me for that final, ultimate release.

He dropped his face to mine, mouth meeting mouth, blocking the view of the others. But I knew they were there. Our tongues mingled. My hips rose to meet his. My back arched. Heat flooded my spine. I pressed my pelvic area to his as pulsations rocked my body and he spewed forth with unprecedented force, like molten lava from a long-smoldering volcano. Then his penis collapsed and both our bodies went limp. We remained spent and exhausted, his cheek pressed to mine, his hand resting against my thigh.

"My darling," he whispered.

I stroked his cheek and looked upward into the indigo sky, drained, yet curiously content. I felt that we had returned from outer space. The spinning had ceased. There was peace and calm. The insanity of the moment of orgasm had passed.

I turned my head.

Jasmine and Arthur continued their lovemaking, Jasmine on top of Arthur, her small body disproportionate to his compelling mass.

I nudged Kurt, who lifted his head to look in their direction.

Jasmine twisted and turned her body on Arthur's, casting strange shadows against the tiled wall of the pool. Kurt's hand slid over my stomach, resting there for a moment. I felt his breathing quicken as we watched the lovers kiss and roll in the grass.

Kurt kissed my cheek and my eyelids, his hands warm on my hips. Jasmine and Arthur switched positions. He was now on top, looking like an alabaster statue reclining in the moonlight, his muscular body and strong buttocks bobbing about, as he thrust himself into Jasmine.

Kurt moaned and then quickly lowered himself so that his face was between my legs. I was wet and sore. He began to lick me tenderly, with soft touches of his tongue, hungry for the smell and taste of me. He sucked the juices of the aftermath of lovemaking. And then, with a soothing, balming aftereffect, his tongue roamed inside me. I continued to watch Jasmine and Arthur as he, poised over her, stiffened, arched his back and yelled aloud before he collapsed beside her. With Arthur's release, I felt my own final moment of relaxation.

After a few moments of silence, Kurt stood up, tall and Nordic-looking. He stretched and smiled a curious smile of contentment. His eyes rested briefly on Jasmine and Arthur. Then he lowered his hand and helped me up. We stood there with our arms around each other, feeling appeased. We had reached the peak of an undiscovered mountain, and now we were descending with confidence, traveling back to reality, further and further away from surrealistic images and wanton desires.

We walked back to the house, barefoot in the grass, hand in hand, shivering from the coolness of the night air. Just before we went into the kitchen, I turned back for a last look at the twinkling lights in the paper lanterns, to smell the lingering fragrance of the garden. We had been propelled into this dream, swept along by unseen forces, drifting from one wave to another. I felt exhilarated.

"Come, darling," Kurt urged, tugging at my arm. Silently we dressed and collected our belongings and, without a word, we closed the door of the lovely, white minipalace behind us and stepped into the waiting limousine.

As we left the compound, Kurt placed his hand on my knee. I cuddled against him, staring at the lights glittering along the dry hills. My breasts ached from Jasmine's bites. My exhausted body felt in need of rest. "Did this evening really happen to us?" I whispered to Kurt.

"Yes, darling," he answered, brushing my hair from my face. "It really happened."

# Rub-a-Dub-Dub . . .

## UNSIGNED

I had talked to Rick on the phone a number of times before setting the filming date. Each time, a sense of personal connection enlivened what would otherwise have been a dull conversation about administrative details and left me thinking about him long afterward. I liked his voice. As I hung up the receiver that morning, I felt a vague pull of excitement. Not excitement connected with the actual filming we were scheduled to do together, although the anticipation of being on camera always had a rush of its own. Something more than that filled the moment. The strength of the voice, the humor, the enticing sense of someone who was willing to risk speaking the unmentionable. There was no denying that I could not wait to meet him.

And wait I did. I had not yet learned that this man of infinite charm and wit was incorrigibly late. When he finally did arrive at my houseboat in San Diego, film crew in tow—and flowers in hand—my heart beat noticeably faster.

"These will look wonderful on the set," he said as he handed me the flowers. I found myself forcing a smile to my lips to conceal my disappointment. Of course they were for the set and not for me. But as he handed the flowers to me, peering down from his six-foot-two frame with his clear pale blue eyes, I felt as awkward as an adolescent.

"Where should we set this stuff up?" he inquired.

"Back here," I motioned and led them all to the back room where we would soon be mixing innuendo with political affairs.

The entourage consisted of one cameraman, who was tall with deep brown eyes hidden behind thick glasses; a sound man, who was short and scruffy, as if he had been working for days without sleep; and Ben, the associate producer, lean, blond and goodlooking—almost too good-looking in the classical sense. And while I found myself viscerally attracted to Rick, Ben was clearly the better-looking of the two. With a tall slim body and finely chiseled features, he had the appearance of a man you might easily expect to find in an advertisement for *Playboy*, or Chivas Regal.

As they busily set up, I dressed. "What would go best with the couch?" I mused.

"As director, I'll decide," Rick offered. "I know about things like that; model for me." I found myself blushing, and the warmth of my face spread throughout my body as I coquettishly donned an outfit or two. And as I changed clothes, I had to admit, I looked good, really good. I looked strong, professional, and *very* female. The final decision was easy. I had known from the start that the lavender silk blouse and deep blue wool suit had the right professional yet sensual look. But the process of modeling for him had electrified my body, and the subtle foreplay it provided set the tone for the rest of the encounter.

The feelings seemed to be projected into the repartee of the interview. His questions had an almost seductive ring to them. Were there double entendres, or was I reading into them what I wanted to hear? Meanwhile, I played my role well, answering his queries with style, wit and intelligence.

When the filming ended and the crew packed up to go home, I popped a bottle of champagne. It only seemed right to celebrate. I also wanted to prolong their stay. While I was not willing to make any obvious move, I was certainly willing to set the scene and provide a nudge in the direction I wanted the evening to take. Besides, I knew they had to film the following day and they were not about to fly back to Chicago for the night. But mostly, I just wanted to keep these wonderful men around a little longer.

As the camera and sound men packed up their gear and began their fond farewells, I felt a sense of disappointment wash over me. My fantasy was about to end. But Rick and Ben made no move to leave with them. "No sense in leaving before the bottle is finished," Rick said. "Besides, I noticed you have a hot tub down below."

"I can have it hot in no time," I responded almost before he finished his sentence. The evening was not about to end. In fact, it might be just beginning, with the best yet to come.

Rick echoed my thoughts precisely. "Great. I've heard a lot about California hot tubs," he said. "And it might be just the perfect end to a great day."

It *had* been a great day. The taping had gone far better than expected, and now the sunset was creating the crowning glory with deep pinks, rich purples and golden yellows streaking the sky as we sat around drinking and talking. While waiting for the hot tub to heat up, a heat of quite another kind seemed to build in the room. Then the moon began to rise, a huge, full, orange harvest moon. It was so perfect it was almost trite. I couldn't have asked Mother Nature to participate more fully. And had Rick not, at that point, offered me a joint, I would have sworn that the beauty of the moment was already drug-induced.

We each inhaled deeply as we passed the joint around. Any stresses of the day seemed to dissolve into a mellow, warm sensuality, the quiet kind of turn-on that warms the body slowly as opposed to the quick rush that accompanies actual lovemaking. A silky thread of expectation glided beneath the conversation. My mind was moving on ahead. How could I communicate my interest without appearing too forward? And what could this mean to my professional reputation and political career? However, sensuality took precedence and propriety plummeted out of sight as I wandered outside, removed the hot tub cover and checked the temperature. "I think it's about time," I called back inside, pulling us out of our reverie. And with champagne and joint in hand, Ben and Rick joined me outside. The moon, which was rising higher in the sky, had turned a translucent silver and was casting a light that illuminated the outlines of our bodies as we slowly removed our clothes. Piece by piece the three of us undressed individually and yet in unison. Not the kind of undressing that blatantly smacks of sexuality, but a subtle sensual dance of beautiful bodies in motion portending a visual taste of what might be in store.

Then, one by one, we slipped the silver-edged luminescence of our naked bodies into the steamy water. With Rick on one side and Ben seated across, I leaned back against the pulsing jet stream of water, closed my eyes and let the strong smooth bubbles massage reality away. It really didn't matter what would transpire. This moment in itself was wonderful.

Suddenly, I sensed an arm casually brush against my shoulder ever so lightly. The nuance of contact sent a rush of energy throughout my body. The imperceptible touch was much more sensual than firm, direct contact. Was it intentional or just a chance movement? I decided to return the gesture by gently sliding my hand along Rick's forearm. Just the barest of touches; it could so easily be accidental. But the electricity betrayed its true intent and Rick responded by caressing my side down to the small of my back. The caress was so light it left me yearning for more. And I was not disappointed. We alternated back and forth, in soft, subtle, teasing motions. We traced the outlines of each other's bodies, moving from the safe areas of back, arms, shoulders and thighs to the curves of our buttocks and into the creases of more sensitive parts. All of this was undisclosed beneath the bubbles from the jets which masked the underwater dance. However, even with the security of the diaphanous curtain that veiled our tentative but tantalizing activities, I wondered about Ben. Did he sense what was going on? Would he discover us? Would he feel left out?

The moon was now high in the dark clear sky. A more perfect evening could not even be imagined. None of us wanted to leave the tub and curtail the beauty of the evening, and certainly I wanted to continue the half-formed dreamlike movements that made promises of more intensity to come. But the water had become unbearably hot. I decided to turn off the heat, and as I did, the security of the bubbles ceased also. The still, clear water made every underwater movement visible, and I feared it would mark the end of our surreptitious tantalizations.

To my surprise, Rick continued as if the full moon did not give perfect access to our manual meanderings beneath the crystal-clear water. I closed my eyes, and like an ostrich who puts his head in the sand, I denied reality. Besides, Ben is Rick's friend, I mused. He and Rick would have to work it out. Meanwhile, Rick's feather-light touches raised goosebumps all over my arms, legs, breasts and buttocks, even in the stifling hot water.

As my body languished in the silent physical exchange of the give-and-take teasing we had been involved in, I thought I perceived some new movement in the water. When I opened my eyes, I could see that Ben had changed his position slightly and was stroking Rick's outer thigh. When Ben began to stroke my thighs as well, I knew that this evening would have more in store than I ever anticipated. As I drifted in that secure and sensual space that only grass, hot water, and the loving attention of two beautiful men can possibly create, my mind entered a semidreamlike state. It was all so natural that I found myself wondering how many times these two men had shared each other in the past. Certainly many experiences had been necessary to develop such a comfortable and loving exchange.

I relaxed my head along the rim of the hot tub and allowed my legs to float up outstretched. As I did so, Rick slowly and delicately began to cup one breast. The soft, almost imperceptible contact of his hands running over the water next to my body made me moan with wanting and desire. My whole being was literally vibrating with tension. I could feel my body lift almost out of the water in an attempt to get closer to them, to take the exquisite teasing one step further, longing for the pressure that just eluded me. Then Rick, while lovingly stroking my breasts, took my taut nipple in his mouth, and as he sucked, currents of excitement shot through me. And when Ben began to suck on my other nipple, I truly found myself wondering if heaven could really be better.

With all of our intentions so clearly out in the open, our hands could roam freely. I traced the creases of both men's inner thighs simultaneously. Rick reciprocated by tracing mine while Ben began to explore the softness of my cunt. I wanted him inside me so badly that I could barely stand it. I felt completely stretched, almost at the breaking point. Rick found my clit, Ben put his fingers inside me, and as I moaned, consumed with desire, my breathing became hard and fast. Within seconds I felt myself expand, beyond the limits of my body, and all at once, an explosion of exquisite force rocked my body into spasm after spasm.

I had never before come so quickly, and with so little touching, yet I was far from satisfied. I hungered for more. And as if in a fantasy, where every wish is instantly fulfilled, the stroking, sucking and loving continued.

I groped for their penises. They were strong and hard. And with the water as a magical silky lubricant, I took one in each hand and with loving gentleness, I stroked up and down, up and down, as they continued to play with my breasts, my cunt, my clit, my ass. Four hands and two mouths saturating my senses and drowning my body into wave upon wave of pleasure. As the tension mounted, one orgasm just seemed to lead to the next until finally, after every nerve and muscle in my body had exploded and convulsed more intensely than I had ever before experienced, I could stand it no more. My clitoris felt excruciatingly tender as if tiny needles were pricking it everywhere and all at once. My body began to contract, away from all the stimulation, and I laughed as I cried out, "Time out!" They laughed, too, as we hugged each other in a way that good friends do when they haven't seen each other in a long time or when one has done something completely delightful or endearing to the other. Then I turned the heat back on so we could remain in the tub a while longer.

Meanwhile, with time to reflect, I noticed the return of that uneasy feeling gnawing at the pit of my stomach. I *was* worried about what others might think. I began fantasizing about newspaper headlines that read "CONGRESSIONAL CANDIDATE'S ILLICIT MÉNAGE" and the copy about how I seduced these men just hours after meeting them. Even in a progressive city, it would deal the deathblow to any possible election. However, when I did let them know my fears, their warm, loving response left me free of concern. "We don't kiss and tell," said Ben. And corny as it was, it made me feel secure.

"Tell me the truth," I inquired. "How many times have you done this before?"

I was shocked by their response. "Never," they said almost in unison. I found it hard to believe, as they were so at ease and completely natural with each other. Yet the conversation that ensued was totally believable. I had no reason to question their response. Both were quite straight, which clarified why, although they were warm and loving with each other, neither ever touched the other genitally. This, of course, meant only more attention toward me, which I certainly wasn't complaining about. Clearly it seemed that their foremost desire was to totally satisfy me. And while Rick had been involved with two women once, Ben had never had a sexual experience that included more than one other person. Yet they were clearly relaxed—and while I had been involved with two men a few times in my life, the fully relaxed and incredibly caring exchange had taken this experience even beyond my most wonderful fantasies.

Finally, after talking and playing around some more, we began to worry that our prunelike skin would never return to normal. Slowly we got out of the tub, the droplets of water glistening in the moonlight. With two towels we took turns lovingly patting down the skin of the third. Fluffy towels gently caressing the necks, shoulders, chests and backs. Probing under arms, around genitals, the creases of the inner thigh and buttocks. As one kneeled to draw a towel over legs and feet, the other caressed the moisture from the face as if we were doing a well-rehearsed dance. After drying each other off, we went into the kitchen. Four hours had elapsed since we first entered the tub. I couldn't remember a more enjoyable period of time.

After nibbling at some cheese and crackers, we walked, still naked, into the living room. We sprawled over the couch. They were draped against the side cushions, their legs crossing to cover my lap as I sat in the middle, and we talked about our lives. Even after such intense sex and intimacy I had no idea that both Rick and Ben were divorced. One lived on Lake Michigan and the other near the university. Their friendship had grown out of the two years they had worked together on a number of documentaries. I shared that I was also divorced and had even spent a few years in Chicago while attending law school. The next few hours were spent filling each other in on our thirty-odd years while we stroked each other affectionately. Our hands wandered around each other's bodies, as carelessly as one might drum his fingers on a table while his mind was elsewhere.

Imperceptibly our talking decreased and our touching increased. I had moved over securely snuggled in Ben's arms while Rick massaged my feet. Ben leaned his face down and kissed me gently. I reacted with an overwhelming sexual energy that should have been more than depleted by now. I slid farther down the couch and put Ben's cock in my mouth, and Rick moved over, kissing my back as he draped his chest and stomach around my buttocks, his knees on the floor. I reached down and slid my hand smoothly along Rick's penis, using his oily secretions to lubricate my hand. Again, my body was filled with pleasure as they both attended to me fully, my sense of touch so heightened that a million light fingers sent pulsing sensations of pleasure throughout my body. As I tried to return their favors, they only teased me by letting me play with their wonderful cocks briefly before drawing back and again concentrating on me. Tension mounted as we moved back and forth and in a variety of positions as if in a ritual dance rehearsed over centuries.

The teasing and touching electrified me until my body was crying out inside, longing to be filled. I was bent over the couch, my legs dangling toward the floor, Rick's cock in my mouth as he lay below me, when Ben began to enter me from behind. His satin softness expanded my interior as if inhaling the deep subtle fragrance of a flower.

"Damn!" I jolted out of my reverie. "I need my diaphragm!"

"Don't move, I'll get it," said Ben as he rose to his feet. "Just tell me where it is."

"Up next to my bed in the ceramic-covered container. And if you don't mind, would you also bring me my robe hanging in my closet and some socks out of my top drawer? I'm starting to feel a bit cold."

"No problem," he said and ran off only to return moments later with diaphragm, cream, robe and a pair of red woolen socks in hand.

"Will these do?" he asked as he handed me the robe and began to unroll the socks. "They looked interesting."

"Wow. They sure do," said Rick as the robe fell to the floor and he concentrated on slipping one sock over one foot and up the leg while Ben did likewise with the second one. They were the above-the-knee kind of socks, and, somehow, sitting on the couch, spreadeagled, wearing only red woolen socks to midthigh was sexier than a black negligee. Rick remained on his knees, stroking my legs and kissing my thighs above the socks, while Ben put the cream into the diaphragm. While stroking himself with one hand, he carefully inserted the diaphragm with the other.

"I'm impressed," I said, joking. "Where did you learn how to do that?"

"I was married once," he replied as he turned me on my side and kneeled so he could enter me from behind again without interrupting Rick's licking and caressing. Then he carefully slipped inside me. "You had to do something to keep sex interesting."

Well, fingers are one thing, but a firm cock is quite another. And as Ben moved gracefully in and out, Rick began kissing me passionately full on the lips, exploring the inside of my mouth, and rolled my nipples between his fingers in an excruciatingly sensitive way. I stroked his cock with the same rhythm orchestrated by Ben's thrusting. We moved as if we were one, building, expanding, moaning, until we reached a peak of sensation and exploded together. Finally the intense spasms and contractions passed as our bodies melted with relaxation and our breathing returned to normal.

Sated and exhausted, we went upstairs to the bedroom to sleep, with me, as had become our style, in the middle. The night was spent with gentle arms affectionately wrapped one around the other, our legs entwined. When we awoke, the sun was high in the sky. We all felt rested, and, since their next shoot wasn't until the evening, we decided to take a drive and visit the zoo. With the top down, the three of us squeezed into the front seat, again with me in the middle. I felt as if I were snuggled between two of my dearest friends, and yet we had known each other less than a day.

We stopped in a small town to eat. With the three of us walking arm in arm down the street, I couldn't help but grin. Rick picked up on it right away. "There goes Gina with her boys," he said with a gleam in his eye.

"You're right," I replied, totally unabashedly. "I may never have this opportunity again in my life, and I'm going to enjoy it thoroughly."

"So are we," he replied. And they both gave me an affectionate squeeze.

# Evesdropping

UNSIGNED

Still half asleep, I open my eyes. The streets are heavy with middle-of-the-night stillness; what could have awakened me? As I stir in bed, I notice that my body is hot, my face flushed. I must have been having a sexy dream.

I turn toward Steve. Curling into his wide back, I try to settle into the way we have of sleeping that we like to call spooning. (When I am in front with Steve behind, I really do feel as if we were two spoons nestled comfortably together, Steve's hand wrapped around me and carelessly cupping my breast. But this way, with me in the back, it doesn't feel like spoons at all. Steve is too big to wrap around.)

I know Steve won't wake up. In the two years we have lived together, we were never both awake in the middle of the night. Steve is an incredibly sound sleeper, probably part of his being twenty-one years old: he falls asleep quickly and wakes up with a smile. I am not so easily satisfied.

I remember the night Steve and I met, a cool starry night at the beginning of our sophomore year in college. We sat on the steps outside the student union and chatted—what could we have said, making small talk as our hearts raced?—and somehow we both ended up a few endless blocks away, upstairs, in Steve's room. Those first kisses of ours were tender, exploring. As I think about them now, I can feel myself blushing over those kisses—so naïve, and yet so hungry. They were deeper and more confusing than any kisses I'd ever known before. Slowly, Steve helped me onto his narrow bed. When he unbuttoned my blouse, running his fingertips up and down my chest, my skin prickled in anticipation. When his opened hand, flat against my belly, found its way inside my panties, I arched my back to meet him with an urgency that surprised me.

Since then, so much has happened. Steve and I have lived together in two different apartments—first with three of his male housemates, and now with the woman who was my best friend during our freshman year, Eve. Steve and Eve, I used to joke—you sound like a vaudeville team. People told the three of us not to live together. They were worried that bad feelings would erupt: maybe Eve would be jealous of me and Steve; maybe Steve would be attracted to Eve, or she to him; maybe, maybe. But people didn't know how complicated the arrangement really could be.

I snuggle closer to Steve, open my mouth to breathe in his sweet scent. Years ago, I used to imagine the luxury of making love all night long. I thought it would be an endless feast, coasting from one course to another on a buffet bed arrayed with patterned linens and thick, warm blankets. But for me and Steve, mornings and afternoons seem to be the sexiest times. The magic closeness of the middle of the night is something we have rarely shared. We try to make love only when Eve is away.

I stroke my thigh and ass absentmindedly as I think of Eve. Eve is an acting major, and she's beautiful, her body moving in that slinking, effortless way that comes with years of study. When Eve got the lead in the university's winter production of A Streetcar Named Desire, the three of us—Eve, Steve and I—went out drinking at our college town's closest imitation of a jazz club. We shared lots of beer, and when the music got going we danced. Steve had had enough after a few fast numbers, but Eve and I wanted more. We kept gyrating together like little kids, giggling as we moved our hips and asses in ways we knew were sexy. When a slow dance came on, we stood still, our feet wide apart, staring at each other. Eve was breathing heavily from our earlier dances, and so was I. Finally, in the half light of the dance floor, we moved toward each other. I don't know which of us moved first; it doesn't matter. We opened our arms to each other, hugged each other close, and began swaying to the sultry music. It was like dancing with a man, but better. I wanted desperately for Eve to open her mouth wide and kiss me on the mouth, but that was one move I didn't dare make first.

On the drive home that night, my head thick with beer, I was still turned on. I listened to Eve chatter happily as the seat of Steve's old VW vibrated under my wet crotch. It seemed a long, long drive, and each time there was a rise in the road I felt a deep, easeful buzz in my groin. Mellow orgasms, I thought to myself. When we got home that night, the three of us shared some marijuana before going to bed, and Steve and I couldn't get each other's clothes off fast enough. He knew how hot, how wet, how willing I was to receive him, and when he exploded inside me I felt strangely calm and grateful. I had been aching for something all night, and Steve filled me.

What huge feelings could come from a few casual bumps and grinds from my best friend! What gorgeous sensations in a car ride listening to her high-toned, honey voice! And then, remembering that night, I suddenly piece it all together. The voice! Eve's voice. It was Eve's voice that roused me from sleep just moments ago.

As I remember, I hear the voice again. Eve is whispering to someone, and it is two o'clock in the morning.

I turn from Steve to listen better. The apartment's two bed-

rooms are separated only by a thin wall, so it is easy to hear.
Eve is talking to a man. Could it be Frank, the dark, handsome
lead in her production? Eve has been talking about him a lot
recently. And though I never met him, I am sure my guess is
right: the male voice that answers Eve's is just the pitch, just
the tone, just the heaviness that comes from acting.

"I don't know," Eve's soft voice is saying. "Try a little higher."

I hold my breath, awaiting the next words. They're his:
"Your skin is so soft. Delicious." Eve giggles.

Then the giggle stops, and Eve begins to breathe more
heavily. Is it her acting training that makes each breath so
loud? I think in annoyance. I feel as though I can see it all:
Frank bent over Eve's smooth thighs, lapping at her genitals
with the tiny smacking sounds that resound in my dark bedroom. And there is Eve, beautiful Eve, on her back, her legs
open wide, her chest heaving in great sighs as her body swells.
It has been a long time since Eve has made love to anyone,
and her sounds go right through me. They are such ecstatic
sounds.

As Eve's breathing grows more urgent, my body reacts as
though it were I who was being eaten. Eve is nearly singing
now. "Oh, God. Oh, God," she calls out in that high, sweet
voice. My thighs and pelvis are hot; so are my cheeks, and
my heart beats so loudly I think it might wake Steve. I move
a little more toward my side of the bed and listen.

A little later, the pitch changes. "Yes, oh yes, yes." She
stretches the "s" sound until it burns in my throbbing head,
and almost without thinking I cup my own hand around my
genitals. I begin to rub.

Eve's words turn to moans. "Ummm, ummmm," and the
pitch deepens even more. Then Frank joins her, moaning too.
"Ummmm, ummmmm." I thrust one finger into my vagina and

marvel at its wetness. I bring the finger to my face so I can smell it—this must be what Eve's smelling like, I think—and I send it back again.

Suddenly, Eve starts grunting. Can humans really make such sounds? The bed squeaks, and I know what is happening: Frank is astride Eve's pert limber body, thrusting his penis deep into her.

I give in to my hot sensations. I rub the mound of my genitals with my hand, feeling my own pulsations deepen as Eve's grunts continue. Gently, I touch my clitoris through my skin. With my eyes closed, I imagine Eve with a faceless, sexy stranger astride her. I picture the expanse of her belly, and the dark hair curling below. My own hand starts rubbing faster, faster, making round luscious circles with little lapping sounds of my own. The pulsing in my groin is constant now, deep, and there's no turning back. The welcome warmth of an orgasm spreads from my genitals to my thighs. The beat of my own hand slows, and the orgasm melts slowly away. My chest is glistening with sweat. I touch my nipples with my other hand, circling round and round. I have another orgasm, smaller this time, and I think some more of Eve and the darker, firmer nipples on her firm breasts.

Suddenly it's Frank's turn. I am startled to hear him groan as throatily, as lusciously, as Eve did. His rich moaning goes straight to my head. I thought only women sounded like that as they came.

I stick a finger in my asshole and feel it pulse, pulse, pulse . . . rapidly and then, as the rooms get quiet, slower and slower still. It's silent now. Frank has come, Eve has come, I have come. I snuggle into Steve again and drift off to sleep.

My dreams are troubled. Eve and I are ice-skating, swirling happily around the college rink, when four men in black leather jackets and slicked-back hair come onto the ice. They skate four abreast, clasping hands by crossing their arms in front of them, and Eve and I are unable to pass. "What are they saying?" Eve asks in dismay.

And then I am awake once more. It's Frank who wakes me this time; he is mumbling again, whispering earnestly to Eve, and she laughs her high crystalline laugh. Then they are making love again. How much time has passed? I wonder. How can he be hard again so soon?

This session is stormier than the first time. I think they have forgotten that there are people asleep in the next room. The whispers aren't whispers now, but throaty sounds yearning to project into full-voiced speech. "I want to be on top this time," I hear Eve say. The bed creaks a little, and I imagine the scene again: Eve upright, her legs tucked beneath that ass, sitting tall so Frank can stroke her beautiful firm breasts. I see Eve arch her back, forcing Frank's hands down her bare belly, following his hand with her own, stroking her skin with a touch both sure and tender.

Eve's moans are deeper, more urgent, coming not from her throat or chest but from her very soul. But it is Frank's moaning that is almost more than I can bear. What does he look like? I see him with a black beard, a black shock of hair, black hair curling down his flat abdomen and around his erect penis. I see him bathed in sweat, stinking through his raw feelings, hard, hard. I see him with his eyes closed, his mouth open, his tongue wet.

No words escape either of them, just animal sounds—hers high-pitched, his low.

Now my body betrays me. It melts again, longing to be in Eve's bed with her and Frank. My hands aren't needed this time. I just lie in my own sweat, feel my ass and my crotch join in a wide-mouthed pulsing of pleasure. "No," I think to myself. "I will not lie here and masturbate again. And I will not lie here and envy Eve." But it is too late. The waves come, on their own. I have again drunk from the banquet Eve and Frank have spread.

When my body cools, I feel terribly alone. Now and again I hear Eve whisper—real whispers this time, not the grunting tones of a half hour ago. Why is no one here with me?

I try to awaken Steve. I stroke his massive back, cup his ass in my hands, rub my genitals against the hard small spot where his back and buttocks meet. Then I reach around his hips and stroke his penis. It is already almost hard—a dream of his? I kiss his shoulders.

Steve rolls toward me, his eyes still closed. "Noisy tonight, aren't they?" he whispers. I kiss his mouth; it's heavy with sleep.

"I feel like I've been awake all night," I say. "Can you just hold me for a while?"

Steve wraps me up and squeezes. His legs and mine entwine, his penis easing its way toward my vagina. I take his penis and tickle my clitoris with the tip. I don't really want him inside me but I want to make him hard. Do I need to show myself that I can? I move my face down to Steve's penis, slowly tracing my route with my fingertips, and take his penis in my mouth. This is the taste I love. As I suck, he grows harder. Steve strokes my hair. I still suck, and suck, and find myself thinking: Frank's penis is like this but bigger. Frank's penis is bigger. Frank's penis has been in Eve's vagina tonight.

I sigh. I'm surprised by how troubled my sigh sounds.

"Oh, baby," Steve says gently. He pulls my shoulders up, places me on his chest and hugs me. "Does it bother you to hear them fucking?" he asks. I grunt in assent. "Don't let it, baby," he says. "Don't let it." I hug Steve and slide off his chest. Curled into myself now, my arms wrapped protectively around my own belly, soon I am sleeping, too.

# ANONYMOUS SEX

## Women Who Love Men Who Love Horses

*SUSAN BLOCK*

She didn't have the time or energy to notice the rough seductive smiles and hard curves of other men. She was too busy
interviewing them, getting them to tell her their deepest, truest,
most personal stories for a study she was doing on personal
ads. Oh, sometimes they'd get a little carried away. After
confessing their most joyous or painful experiences to an open,
attractive woman such as she, in an intimate setting such as a
bar or their bedroom, they'd naturally wish to make love to
her. After all, since she possessed their secrets, they wanted
to possess her.

But she was never tempted. She considered them all subjects
for her study, fuel for her imagination. And every Thursday
night at midnight, no matter what city she was in, when she
called David, she could always say "I miss you" with an utterly
clear conscience. He never asked if she was "unfaithful"; they
didn't use words like that.

She was looking forward to her next stop—New Haven, a
town where she'd spent four of her wildest, most promiscuous
years. That was the way college tended to be, even a stuffy
old school like Yale.

When she reached the hotel, there was a message waiting
for her. It was from one of her New Haven subjects, whose
personal ad went something like:

SWM, athletic, attractive, heir to multimillion-dollar for-
tune, would like to meet Yalie who loves men who love
horses.

It was what she called one of those "too-good-to-be-true" ads
that had to have a hitch. His wanting a "Yalie" made her
suspicious; her old alma mater had academic power, but very
little sex appeal. Then again, "Yalie" could mean "man" or
"woman"; there was no telling with the personals.

The "horse" part intrigued her, though. She hadn't ridden
since she was eight, at the zoo, but images of ancient, mythical
centaurs—half men, half horses—stampeded through her
dreams, often waking her in the night. She'd sit up with a
start, ready to ride off with them, disappointed to be left
behind. She was looking forward to this interview. She wanted
to know what he'd found out about women who loved men
who loved horses.

"A Mr. Aaron Van der Tak," the hotel desk clerk was saying,
"called to confirm your interview for Thursday at noon at his
estate. He asks, 'Can you do interviews on horseback?'"

Sure, she found herself saying out loud, she could do interviews in helicopters, hot tubs, anywhere they liked.

Fortunately, all five Wednesday interviewees met her in the
hotel café. By midnight, she was exhausted, filled to over-
flowing with other people's love stories. But the relentless
thump-a-thump from the hotel disco on the floor above her
kept her wide awake for hours, envisioning couples in skin-
tight jump suits bumping and grinding, laughing and flirting,
dancing down the halls into each other's beds. Maybe they'd
break into her room, force themselves on her, dancing all over
her. She shivered with disgust and terror, then sat up and
stared at her locked door, worrying that these long months

without David were turning her into a cold observer of other people's passions, incapable of erotic feeling, horrified by the sounds of sexual play. She covered her fears with an image of David hanging upside down from his gravity boots as he did every day after work. She liked to go over to him when he hung like that and hug him around the hips while he hugged her back, nuzzling him between his thighs as he licked the insides of her legs.

She pulled the pillow over her head and cried a little. But not much. She never cried much when she was alone.

On Thursday, rows of apple trees ran through the orchard like golden bracelets. It was his orchard, that is, the Van der Tak family orchard, on the Van der Tak family estate, and she drove past it in her Budget Rent-a-Car just before pulling into the Van der Tak family stable where Aaron—and Aladdin— were waiting for her.

Aaron wasn't her type, of course—too young, too tall, too macho with that arrogant flaming mustache of his. She preferred her men small like herself, sensitive and refined like David. But, in a more objective sense, she supposed he was "attractive." Even somewhat sexy—with the kind of long, endless legs that adorn men's jeans commercials. Though his own jeans weren't the designer kind—they were ripped in both knees—and he stood up to his heels in horseshit. His eyes were what impressed her, bright green like young leaves, like Alan's eyes—her brother.

They introduced themselves. He wiped his hand on his tan work shirt and shook hers. Suddenly, she realized she was wearing all white—white pants, her new white aerobic sneakers, an ivory angel-hair sweater. And as she wondered if maybe she wasn't overplaying the untouchable image, she flipped on her tape recorder.

"So, what made you want to place a personal ad?" she asked. It was her warm-up question.

"Oh, I don't know." He opened the stable door, and a large ebony-colored horse sauntered out. "I guess I'm too shy to just go up and talk to an intelligent, pretty woman. Though I'm talking to you now, aren't I?"

"This is different," she reminded him. "It's an interview."

"Right," he replied, brushing the horse's glistening coat. "Well, we're supposed to do this interview on horseback, aren't we?"

"Oh, sure." She was afraid of this. "Where's the other horse?"

"Oh, Aladdin can take the two of us. He's young, but strong."

"Like you?" she quipped, not imagining he'd blush so.

"I like to ride bareback," he continued. "Aladdin likes it too. You don't mind going without a saddle, do you?"

She shrugged. It was all equally unfamiliar to her. Though that word "bareback" aroused visions of reckless rodeo cowboys on silver steeds bucking and lurching until they fell down hard in the dust.

But Aladdin wasn't silver. He was black with a long white streak plunging from the middle of his forehead to his nostrils, which flared at the odor of humans. His own smell was thick and sweet, dizzying to her unaccustomed senses. To keep her balance, she looked straight into his eye, which was peeking out from beneath his mane. That eye, big as a baby's fist, deep and dark as the earth, stared right into her soul and seemed to say, "Stick with me, babe, we're gonna fly."

She longed to interview this immense, enigmatic animal. She wanted to ask him the secrets of the wild unbridled spirit that galloped countless nights through her dreams.

Aaron pulled two large red apples out of a bag. "Here," he said. "You distract him with these, and I'll slip him into the bit."

Distract him? She contemplated juggling the two fruits in one hand, something her brother Alan had taught her. But such simple tricks wouldn't impress a creature of Aladdin's obvious depth. She thrust out the larger apple for him to examine with his soulful eye, and before she could flinch, he'd chomped the whole thing right out of her palm. His mouth was a frothy mess, he'd dribbled all over her white pants, and Aaron hadn't even appeared with the bit. She resolved to make the second apple last and last. Holding it just beyond Aladdin's reach, she turned it back and forth, letting the sunlight roll around its surface. The horse stepped forward. She stepped back. He snorted, took another larger step, and she offered the apple, pulling it back before he could take more than a tiny bite. He chewed and slurped, his eye catching hers, a warrior's gaze, a challenge. She pulled the apple behind her back and swayed as Aladdin turned his head this way and that, whinnying. She ran backward a few yards, and as soon as Aladdin caught up, she held out the half-eaten apple. He devoured it lustily, his wet lips brushing her palm. She was laughing and shaking the pulp off her pants when Aaron appeared with the bit.

"Okay," he said. "Now distract him with the apples."

Aladdin didn't need to be distracted. He accepted the bit, like a warrior accepting his helmet, his eye on hers. They mounted and took off down the path.

They were flying! They'd been marching and trotting and cantering and then—blast-off through red-gold streaks that used to be trees—they were flying! At least she felt like they were. She recognized the feeling—crazed and breathless—from roller coasters slamming into curves and sparkling waterfalls and sex with David during those wild, romantic first two months. Lately, sex with David wasn't exactly wild; it was tender, loving, good. But not that mad, boundless feeling; they knew each other too well for that. They were far beyond those initial, dizzying, star-smashing marathon sex sessions. Now they made love twice a week more or less. It was restful, comforting, "mature" sex.

But now here was that high-octane feeling again, on a bareback horse through the wind in the fall behind the strong supple back of a millionaire.

"You like to gallop?" he whispered.

"I like to gallop," she said. Her arms clutched his waist. Her legs, now filthy, tightened around Aladdin's flanks, sinking into the moist black velvet of his coat. She was entering her recurrent dream, riding the mythical half man, half horse, the noblest of creatures with the greatest of appetites.

She wondered if David could see her. She imagined him hanging from the branch of an apple tree, watching her, upside down. His eyes were clear and blue as swimming pools. She couldn't tell what they were seeing, but they made her nervous. She hugged Aaron tighter, feeling his warmth through his soft flannel shirt. She didn't care; she was flying through hoops of fire.

"Well, we should trot a little," he said. "So you can interview me."

The red-gold streaks slowed down into trees; their mad flight grounded. Yet her heart still galloped, her thighs jumping with electric charge. Slowing down was the last thing she wanted to do. She wanted to take the reins herself and fly. But she just pushed the damp hair out of her eyes and checked her tape recorder. Aladdin clip-clop-clopped along, his sharp spine cutting into her tailbone.

"Yes, the interview," she repeated. "So . . . tell me . . . about women who love men who love horses."

"You mean tell you what we did together?" He turned, jade

eyes flashing. "But I never talk to a woman about my experiences with other women. They're too jealous."

"Look," she said, "this is my job. And I don't have any reason to be jealous, do I?"

"Oh, well, in that case... Let's see, on my first day, I wore my cowboy boots and tight black pants and nothing else. She was beautiful. We caught the sunset as we rode into the orchard and got the moonrise on the way back. We gave each other massages and took off each other's clothes, piece by piece. She was wearing peach satin panties and those ribbons, you know..."

He went on for over an hour, whispering steamy tales of personal-ad conquests into her ear as her tape recorder rolled and Aladdin trotted along, gently pushing her pelvis into Aaron's million-dollar hips.

The money a man had rarely held much appeal for her. She certainly didn't love David because he paid fifty dollars more rent than she did. Even when a man paid for her lunch, she felt a little uncomfortable, as if she owed him something. But a man with millions—inherited millions—was different. She could let him pay her way without a second thought.

"You want to gallop again?" he whispered like leaves rustling.

"Yes!" She buried her face in the sweet musky smell of his hair. He had freckles on his ears. She felt like kissing them. But didn't. They were off and flying. And then back again.

Her tapes had run out. Her clothes were a mess. She looked at Aaron looking at her on opposite ends of the couch in his "bachelor's pad"—a little guesthouse in back of the Van der Tak mansion. She wondered how *his* ass could take Aladdin's spine. Maybe it had calluses. She didn't ask. *Hers* hurt like hell. He grinned at her and played with the rip in his jeans. She'd felt infinitely closer to him on horseback.

It was just as well. She was getting tired of this sensual

merry-go-round, and she wanted to get a salad or something before going back to the hotel to call David.

But he wanted to show her his snapshot album. He moved closer to her, opening the book across their laps. And in the midst of the mélange of family photos was a shot of Aaron in sweat pants and headgear holding a trophy: "1978 Connecticut State Champion: WRESTLING ." She stared at the picture, superimposing it in her mind over the memory of her brother wearing the same outfit, the same giddy look on his face, holding up the same sort of trophy: "1968: Pennsylvania State Champion: WRESTLING." It was an odd coincidence, causing images to float up of wrestling holds he'd taught her—half nelsons, reverses, cradles—and every other night, when their parents were asleep, they'd go a few rounds on the living room rug. It wasn't much of a contest: he was so much bigger, and he always won. But it was a different kind of game, a special secret rite which they shared at night.

"You like wrestling?" Aaron asked. "Most women don't."

"I—my brother used to wrestle. He taught me—"

"He did, huh?" Aaron shot out of his seat and knelt down on the carpet in the wrestling starting position. "Let's see what he taught you."

She gazed down at the sleek male form waiting for her on its hands and knees. It looked like a horse, ready for her to mount and take off. She giggled at the thought.

"Not up to it, huh?" he said without budging in that jeering, jockish tone just like her brother used when she would chicken out of a challenge. She felt the old sibling dare rush through her, taunting her into the game again. She always knew she'd never win, but she had to play, she loved the ritual, and she hadn't played it in so very long.

She got down on the carpet, grasped his left wrist in her left hand, putting her right arm around his chest. She thought she was holding David for a moment, but was overwhelmed again by the sense of her brother fused somehow with this strange young man whose heart thumped hard against her palm.

"Okay," she whispered.

She pulled his wrist and he turned and pushed and they tumbled into a tangle of holds and escapes. She wrestled with pure abandoned energy, really trying to win this time, to even up old scores between her and Alan, who had beaten her every time. But her opponent was neither gentlemanly nor chauvinist enough to "let the lady win." They rolled around the room, panting and pushing, until there she was, flat on her back, his long strong fingers wrapped around her shoulders, pinning her once again to the carpet.

"Pin," she conceded, her vision doubling with sweat. She looked up into his eyes, green flowers blossoming into Alan's eyes, into the eyes of the centaur who had ridden through so many of her nights.

"Shit," he said hoarsely, "you're strong."

She relaxed upon that benediction. Perhaps she had won after all. Perhaps she had won every time. Perhaps it didn't matter; losing was winning if you knew how to lose, how to transform what you got into what you wanted.

His lips dropped onto her forehead, heavy with exertion, pressing her, pulling her hot skin to his, as their tongues began to wrestle. Her imagination galloped through time, landing on her parents' living room rug with Alan again as their wrestling holds flowed into escapes and caresses. "Yes," she whispered, as she looked up into her brother's emerald gaze, seeing their father and his father and grandfather. "*No!*" she screamed. She shook with terror, but she didn't stop. She wanted to do this, she had to do it, to fly into the center of the forbidden, to learn the secrets, the true difference between body and imagination, the brother and sister within. She kissed him, a long, liquid kiss that rushed through her veins and melted her bones.

"Alan!" she cried.

"No, it's Aaron."

She opened her eyes and saw a handsome young stranger with green eyes. And she relaxed, remembering where she was, remembering Alan, David and all the men she had known, slipping off her clothes one by one as she let each of her trapdoors open. She explored their endless slopes and crevices, a conquistador discovering the City of Gold, the Fountain of Youth engulfing her. They opened the window to her womb, fanning the fire, holding it open with their hands so she could feel the wild horses leap and gallop out of it. Then they galloped in, hot and swift, plunging in, filling her with power. The features of her brother flickered across, then transformed into her wild centaur whisking her over the moon, as Aaron murmured, "Marry me. I want to marry you. I want to be with you every night. . . like this."

They rode on invisible horses in inner space, weightless, timeless, spinning through the dark fog.

She awoke wondering where she was, knowing she needed something in her stomach to help her land on earth. She got up and made grilled cheese sandwiches.

"This is fantastic!" Aaron exclaimed. "You can cook! Now I have to marry you."

She smiled, marveling at how strange and yet how familiar he could be simultaneously.

"Why shouldn't you marry me?" he demanded. "I'm young. I'm handsome. I'm a multimillionaire. And I love you. I can talk to you. I'll do anything for you, and that's no hollow promise because I can afford to do anything for you."

He stood before her, arms outstretched, a golden Apollo, a great tree, offering himself and all of his millions. She felt light-headed again, visions of David springing into her head like jack-in-the-boxes. Suddenly, she remembered, it was Thursday night! Her night to call David. She looked up at Aaron, that glorious banner of youthful maleness, naked and glistening with their mix of emissions.

"Can I use your phone?"

His arms dropped, two falling branches. "Sure," he said, turning away from her.

She pushed the buttons slowly, trying to decide whether she could possibly tell David the truth as she always had, and if not, where to say she was calling from without actually lying to him. A friend's house? Still doing an interview? That was the truth, wasn't it?

"Hello."

"David?"

"No David here." It was her brother's voice. "You got the wrong number—"

"Alan?"

"Yeah. Who's this?"

"Uh . . . your sister."

"What? Oh, hi— Hey, what's up? You all right? Is David—"

"David's fine, Alan. I'm not with David. I've been . . . uh . . . wrestling."

"Wrestling?"

"With the 1978 Connecticut State Champ."

"*Really* wrestling?"

"Really wrestling."

"Did you win?"

"Win?"

"You know what I mean."

"Oh, yeah. Yeah, I won."

"That's my sister."

"Yeah. Well, it's been nice talking—I mean, this is long distance, so—"

"Oh, sure. Well, have fun."

"Okay, I will. See you."

She put down the receiver, amazed at her mistake, and laughed, shaking the images from her head, grabbing her dashing would-be fiancé. She licked the grilled cheese off his lips. She licked his ears, pushing her tongue deep inside until she heard him gasp, and felt him hard against her again. They collapsed on the carpet, knocking over the telephone.

"Tell me," she said, "about women who love men who love horses." His eyes opened wide, jade pinwheels spinning. His head dropped down between her thighs, his tongue moving in slow voluptuous circles, tasting, touching, watering her garden. One flower blossomed inside another inside her—a huge bridal bouquet opening and closing and opening again. The bouquet burst into a thousand water lilies floating on a pond under him, their bodies floating together, wed. He moved in deeper, slow-dancing his wedding dance, like a horse prancing. Then she became the horse, the giant fabled Trojan Horse, and he was fifty men, all her lovers, entering her, filling her up, until she could hold no more, and then they charged through the walls of Troy, exploding the old powers that held her, setting the city on fire, unlocking its ancient secrets, freeing the forbidden answers to her questions.

In the morning, she knew this was her last interview. She kissed Aaron's forehead, silently thanking him as he slept, wishing him well in his search for a wife. Then she put on her not so white clothes and drove off to find a phone to tell David she was coming home.

# The Moon Over SoHo

## UNSIGNED

Take tonight: the two of us are sitting around, having spilled from the hot apartment onto the fire escape, and Frederica goes into her spiel on men. She's a big haughty girl, a New Zealander. If she's to be believed, things are pretty wild down there in Dunedin. You lose your virginity at twelve and after that it's sex with young globe-trotting adventurers—until you're married off in a white lace gown to someone rich, respectable and sheep-owning, of course.

Is Dunedin on the "veldt"? Probably not, but I wonder about it with the damp Manhattan heat beating me to the punch each time I try to think or move. At any rate, I sit there envisioning savanna: it ripples in the rising heat, the sun seizes absolute power over all, zebras swelter in the pathetic shade of the acacias, locusts whine like tiny motors . . . it's all too much. That's how I know I'm drunk.

Cognac, the cocaine of liquors. The taste of that aged oak cask where the amber liquid's lain for God knows how many years underground in a maritime province. I've brought us the best brand, because why not? and also because she'll say, "Oh, Janine, what *lovely* taste." After 1.5 liters, it's no real marvel we're drunk, plastered with our own sweat to the rust of the railings. There's been a record heat wave all week on the eastern seaboard—102 degrees till 2 A.M.—and the city is ripe with all manner of smells that hang in the mayonnaise-like air and rub themselves into your face.

Frederica can outshout anyone, and does, whether they're shouting back or not. Here she is, draped over the fire escape in nothing but a skinny T-shirt and panties, arching and stretching her lithe long legs like a cheetah in heat, and yelling about America. "This country is absolutely *mad*," she pronounces in that distinct accent that must be heard to be believed. (Indeed, how can anyone for a block in every direction *not* hear it?) "And the men! Not even worthy of the name, Lord save them—"

How to get Frederica to shut up when she's in her cups? I'm feeling rowdy but not rowdy enough to subdue her. Below us, meanwhile, this little gang of Puerto Rican youths has been gathering, attracted no doubt by the word "men" if not by the white shimmer of our underwear at the fifth-floor level. They stare upward and laugh at us in Spanglish; one of them puts his hands in his pants and starts squeezing. I'm squatting on my haunches. As I look down between my legs at the youths— who are trying to free the ground-floor fire escape ladder— something tingles and goes Ping! silently, inside my cunt. Suddenly my crotch is wet. I cup it in my hand. Wish one of these guys could shoot his cock up five stories and catch me right there. . . . A low moan slips from my throat as I rub myself a little. The stars are reeling overhead.

Frederica springs onto the outside rail and crouches, a large golden cat. "I've always wanted to do this," she murmurs, pulling aside her panties until her big dark muff is showing. Evidently Frederica is attempting to pee on our audience. I open my eyes in time to see the youths leap back like a fissioning atom. Still not a drop of anything out of Frederica. "Fucking hell, I must be in*hibi*ted." Now the youths, understandably pissed off, are rattling the ladder in earnest. It yields to them. Six angry Hispanics are on their way up to fuck the insolent gringas.

(Earlier this evening we had to vacate the Carmine Street pool under similar circumstances. Frederica showed her breasts to one of the sleazy lifeguards. "He dared me!" she protests as I tried to explain. "Look, these guys are not 'cool' about tits and ass. You'll get into a lot of trouble," etc., etc. No use.)

It's going to be one of those nights.

Getting unsteadily to my feet, I reflect that while Frederica might well imagine she'd enjoy meeting some *real* men for a change, I would just as soon split, have another sip or two of cognac, put on some interesting cosmetics, dress up in a hip outfit and go cruising for guys who are a little more my *type*. . . .

I pull Frederica inside amid her protestations that she can handle herself perfectly well, thank you very much. (It isn't I who've saved her skin, though; the fire escape is busted at the fourth floor so our admirers can't reach us anyhow. They content themselves with howling colorful insults and shaking the entire structure until it seems about to collapse. Frederica moons her ass at them and then we climb back in through the window. Fuck 'em if they can't take a joke.) Myself, I've now returned to swilling cognac in readiness for our next maneuver.

Somewhere past exhilarating midnight, we are headed down Eighth Street to the St. Mark's Bar and Grill, a dark and lucky spot. The East Village streets are packed with people sending out a crossfire of scents, looking for sex, slicing through the air like hot knives through butter. I feel at home in a sensual dream, knowing that soon some sweet-smelling man's swollen cock will be pushing into me.

We're almost to First Avenue and I don't know how we got here. Must have had a blackout—pretty common with cognac. We're in the pink of health, though: we've only been up since 6 P.M., when we hit the pool on Carmine Street; it's way too hot to be moving around in the daytime. Frederica, as you might imagine, walks fast, like a woman striding uphill on skis. I walk normally, I suppose, all things considered.

Men of all shades and shapes are calling to us. "Hey, you're beautiful." "C'mere a minute." "O la la"—yes, one actually says that—"I wanna eat you raw, baby." "Ooh, let's fuck." Can they tell we're ready? It's down to a mere matter of picking the juiciest one. At the thought of that juice, the blood leaves my head and rushes elsewhere. I sway dizzily and bump into this young guy who's been stalking me for three or four blocks now.

"Sorry," I mumble. He just grins and draws his palm slowly across my breasts, his other hand braced in the small of my back. He's a real beauty—about nineteen, muscular and olive-skinned, a big tattoo on his smooth biceps (which he shows me, still grinning), shining brown eyes and curly hair. I almost faint. My mouth opens involuntarily. This is it.

Outside the St. Mark's an overflow crowd is milling purposefully. The flow of events now takes a quantum leap. Frederica has vanished into the whirlpool of predator and prey, and my boy is hailing a cab, thank God. I just want to *do* it. *Now.* "Let's go to my place," I sigh. "Two-hundred block of Spring Street." "Great," says the boy brightly, and we fall into the taxi together. "Two hundred Spring," he tells the cabbie, then starts kissing me enormously up one side of my face and down the other, enveloping lips, earlobes, eyelids in his hot mouth while our hands madly grope for each other's nipples, thighs, bellies and asses like desperate blind creatures. By the time we've traveled the few blocks to Frederica's apartment, my legs are parted wider than the whole back seat and my black velvet skirt is pushed up past my hips to accommodate the huge bulge growing in his pants. The cab lurches to a halt and with unconcealed resentment our driver sneers, "Get outta here." We unpeel ourselves from the back seat and my boy hands the fucker ten bucks.

In the elevator the boy—I think his name's Rick or Ron—sticks a bottle of warm Miller High Life in my mouth. I taste his saliva as I suck. Hey, this boy *understands* women's clothing. In one neat motion he yanks the skirt up again and deftly pops out all four of my garters. He can *tell* that although my black cashmere sweater looks like a pearl-buttoned cardigan, it is to be drawn up over the head. Propped in one corner of the elevator, I throw up my arms as he deftly starts to undress me—the Miller High Life goes smash in a spray of glass and foam. The bra's a little harder but he undoes that, too, and buries his face in my cupped breasts while I reach behind myself to pull my panties down.

They've no sooner dropped to the floor than his cock is probing for the wet lips of my cunt. At the sight of it, long, glistening, purple-veined, smooth as rosy silk, I groan loudly, it's so beautiful. I can't wait to feel it penetrate me: it's been a whole day since I fucked last, after all. By now my French twist has fallen around my face in a cascade of sweat.

How long has the elevator been at Frederica's floor? Still the hard gleaming head of the boy's penis is rocking against my parted labia, butting quickly in and out but in no hurry to take the plunge. I'm dying. His teeth and tongue strafe one nipple as his hand kneads the other. The cock sticks out of his jeans like a slightly bent arrow, aimed so high he has to bend sharply at the knees, giving me a little taste, then withdrawing it. Exquisite torture. My groans may turn to screaming any moment.

The door glides open and in step the nice squat middle-aged Nicaraguan couple who live next door to Frederica. They step back out just as fast. To their credit, they don't even titter. But their appearance is enough to kick my boy into action. Grasping my thighs around his waist, he hoists me onto his loins. *In* like a bolt slides his cock. Ecstasy. But I can't move, I can't even squirm, I'm locked in a tight embrace as he brushes past the Nicaraguans and down the hall. (Farewell forever to my sweater and panties. What was I wearing a sweater for, anyway? Too fucking hot for a sweater.)

"It's this one," I murmur at the door of 515, my face nuzzling his scalp and temples. "The key's on the lintel." (Believe it or not some guys have to ask what a *lintel* is. Not this one.) He reaches up with his hard tattooed arm and grabs the key and we're in.

The room is glowing faintly in the glare of New York night. Stars, neon, office fluorescence, sodium and mercury vapor, the full moon, Grand Opening searchlights, floodlit corporate plazas, a million blue TV tubes—their rays steam and mingle with the rhythm of a far-off Latin station, the low drone of the building air conditioner, the scent of the lavender oil Frederica added to her bath, the rush of traffic. My mattress lies by the open window, a single crumpled sheet and pillow on it. Slowly the boy sinks to his knees and tips me backward onto the bed, never taking his eyes off my cunt. "Now we're gonna fuck," he moans, as if from deep sleep. "We're gonna make love." His jeans and T-shirt are off him; my nylons are still held by my strapped-on heels. Where did my skirt go? Who cares?

Rapidly he wipes the sweat and my juice from his cock. Laying his palms on the insides of my thighs, he forces my legs apart as far as they'll spread. I can't take my eyes off that beautiful penis. Then I have to, because he starts to thrust hard and fast, his round balls slapping my flesh, his hands convulsively squeezing my breasts. These are pushed up as far as they'll go and thrilling with the burn and tickle of sex that jets from my cervix to the roof of my mouth. I'm panting and gasping, thrusting back and kissing his penis hard with my vagina. As soon as my whimpers reach a certain pitch, the boy slips it out, wipes away the sweat that's trickled down his creamy chest to his belly, then enters me again, and again and again.

I can see how this boy's cock must have gotten bent: when he thrusts he doesn't aim, he just lunges until it's in up to the hilt. When he rolls me over and tries to ram it up my ass, though, my whimpering becomes a sharp cry of pain. I'm not tight, but nature does have its limits. . . . Gripping me by the hips and jacking my ass upward, he changes angle and rams it up my cunt instead, all the way to the cervix. "Just like animals," he croons in that weird drugged voice. I find I can rock against him as hard and fast as I want to; this guy's not going to quit pumping till I can't come anymore.

Yellow light from the hall falls across us as Frederica and a tall black man stumble into the apartment. "Aw, gimme a fuckin' break!" protests my boy. "Don't stop!" my voice breathes, muffled from the sweaty sheet. "They're friends—of mine—" From the corner of my eye I see the man gazing cynically at us. He's already stripped to the waist, a pale leather jacket over his arm. He looks like a bitter-chocolate god.

My boy is watching, too, all the while digging deep between the splayed cheeks of my rump, now staccato, now glissando, stroking my breasts and sometimes snaking his hands down to play with both pairs of my lips. Without a word, Frederica and her lover strip. Our spasms hit a new, involuntary plane: I couldn't have imagined us becoming more aroused than we are already, but the sight of Frederica kneeling to suck the guy's mounting hard-on does it. Her golden thighs are quaking with excitement.

By this time I'm coming in a nonstop hysterical stream, the ache of penetration shuddering all through me. I bite the pillow and grip the mattress edges for dear life. The black very deliberately opens the refrigerator, peers into it disdainfully, then takes out something I can't see. Sliding his dick out of Frederica's greedy throat, he lathers himself with whatever he found in the fridge. "Pussy," he hisses. Apparently Frederica understands this cryptic remark, because she rises in stately fashion to her feet and twists around into a low bend over the bathtub; her rump arches, two round white mounds. She's "presenting"—there's no other word for it. Somehow the black man manages to distance himself from that tempting display. He lays only one black hand on the whiteness and by centimeters forces that long black cock up her ass.

Frederica is caressing her own stiff breasts and their rosettes, making noises in the back of her throat. Mouth wide open, half groan, half cough, it's like the chuffing of a lioness in estrus. She surrenders to convulsions. "You—bastard—you— bastard—you—bastard—" she groans. My boy is like a rock, his balls are hard bristling peaches full to bursting. In a blaze of bliss I find myself wanting them to burst at last.

I brush the sweaty hair from my eyes and look: the black is lathering his left hand now, the right still resting on Frederica's soft white ass. The boy hugs me even tighter and bites into the back of my neck. The black returns my stare with cold contempt. And with his dark cock ramming in and out of Frederica's ass, he guides several black fingers into her cunt. My boy takes one look, "Aaaaaaaahhhhhhhh!" erupts out of him and he comes, hot and wet, as only a virile teenager can. We collapse in exhaustion. A pool of semen seeps out onto the bed.

"You *bastard*," roars Frederica. She loves it. A cock in her ass, a hand up her tight little cunt. But with a jerk the black pulls out of her. Frederica gradually swivels about and lunges on the rim of the bathtub, surveying him with ice-blue eyes. Roughly but methodically he steps into his clothes, and stalks to the door. A parting shot—"Fucking white bitch"—then he's gone.

"*Quite,*" giggles Frederica, massaging her moist behind. She darts a hungry speculative look in our direction but perhaps she senses I wouldn't welcome her into my bed at the moment. Stretching extravagantly, she saunters to the ladder and vaults up onto her makeshift bunk.

The boy is in some kind of exalted state which I don't care to investigate. "You make love real good," he breathes. I murmur something in return. He kisses me with reverence. For the last time I feel his downy cheek on mine. "Good night, Rick," I whisper, already drifting off. "It's Ron," he says, smiling sweetly.

# A Very Special Dance

## CAROL CONN

The heavy, sweet smell of incense envelops me as I enter the reggae club alone. The music has started and the audience sways in their chairs to the hypnotic tempo. I wander around greeting friends and acquaintances. One offers me a line of coke, another shares some Jamaican grass.

Soon I am high, and the music transports me to another dimension. Reggae bass penetrates my nervous system, each beat pulsating deeper and deeper into my spine.

Ah, release, body loosens as each joint and limb lets go of tension. Arms flow like scarves billowing in a gentle breeze. Hips shimmy and dip in slow undulations. Shoulders move unto themselves, fluid and lithe as an ocean wave.

Mind gradually sheds all anxieties, worries and cares. Responsibilities cease to matter. My whole being is tuned to the music.

I am now on the dance floor, swaying with the crowd. My thoughts are not with the lesbians to my left, Rasta groupies in front, or the attractive black couple to my right. I am completely absorbed in my own free movements. A direct communion with the music. Ecstatic prayer.

The crowd has swelled, the air now steamy. A fine sheen of perspiration coats my body, from the pores on my scalp to the growing moistness between my legs. The beat continues, lulling me further into a sensuous state of relaxation. The dance floor is so crowded that arms, hips and hands softly bump into others nearby.

There is a different feel to whoever is behind me. I can't tell if this dancer is a man or woman. I am too entranced in the music to turn around. Occasionally a knee softly grazes my ass, a hand brushes my hip. Hypnotic as the music is, this dancer invades my soporific state. I move forward to escape but the careless feet of the groupies in front of me force me back.

I stumble backward, feel a hard swelling and know that it is a man. I turn slightly, but my hip undulations keep me rubbing up against his erection. My body starts to crave the contact as my back, hips and ass become more attuned to the stranger's movements. His hands guide my hip gyrations as we dance in near-perfect synchronism.

Now my heart skips a beat each time my ass or hips meet him. His hands remain on my hips, gradually pulling me closer until I can feel his chest touch my shoulders, belt buckle in my spine. The music keeps me there. I don't panic because the touch, feel, even the smell of this stranger is so familiar.

His hands stroke my breasts, nipples rigid under fingertips. A lucid moment of fear briefly sets in. But I notice that everyone is totally into the music and oblivious to the surroundings.

The stranger lulls me back into his sphere. I yield to his soft strength. His arms encircle me and we sway to the music as one. My hips automatically respond, pushing back into him. Farther, farther.

Somehow his hand has moved discreetly under the loose folds of my black gauze skirt. He easily slides my panties down and his fingers begin a slow massage in time to the music. He matches each chord of the powerful bass with a deep thrust. My only fear now is that the music will climax before I do. The suspense builds and builds. The music is endless.

I am quivering, breathless and hot.

Instinctively I arch my buttocks and grind against his pelvis. He teases me until I moan. The tension is too much. I turn my head slightly but can only glimpse a beard streaked with gray in the dim light.

It doesn't matter. I now know who he is.

Never taking his fingers from my throbbing clit, he takes my breath away, making me gasp. A cold fire spreads, leaving me suspended on an endless edge. I dissolve into a paroxysm of explosions, his body pulsating in unison.

My knees go weak. He catches me as I am about to fall, holding me up until I can recover my balance.

The set ends and the crowd goes wild. I limply clap my hands and turn to kiss this kind partner. Small thanks for such a memorable dance.

# BIOGRAPHIES

**Carolyn Banks's** novels include *The Girls on the Row, Mr. Right* and *The Darkroom.* She is a reviewer for the Los Angeles *Times* and the Washington *Post* and has had feature articles in *Sports Illustrated, American Education, Family Weekly, Redbook* and others. Her short stories have appeared in *American Mix, In Youth* and other anthologies. She is presently working on a screenplay.

**Lonnie Barbach** is a clinical psychologist and author. In addition to numerous articles in professional journals and chapters in academic books, she has published in *Ladies' Home Journal, Mademoiselle, Ms., Self, Cosmopolitan, Glamour, Playgirl, Brides* and others. She is the author of *For Yourself, For Each Other* and *Women Discover Orgasm* and coauthor of *Shared Intimacies* and *The Intimate Male.* She won honorable mention in the American Medical Writers Award, and has created an educational self-help video on female sexuality.

**Susan Block** is the author of *Advertising for Love,* a book about the personal ads. She writes freelance for a number of magazines, including *Playgirl, Oui,* the *L.A. Weekly* and *Los Angeles Magazine.* She is also a published poet, an as yet unproduced screenwriter, a produced playwright, an actress and director and the writer-performer of *Mattress Madness,* a one-woman show with clean sheets.

**Wickham Boyle** wears two hats. She is president of a small management consulting company, City Specials, and is also a writer. She is the author of *On the Streets: A Guide to New York City Buskers,* an anecdotal compendium of street performers. She is the author of *Alice in Numberland,* a satirical look at women in business schools. She has written articles about rowing, carpentry and growing up or not and is currently at work on a series entitled *Dances with My Father.*

**Carol Conn** is a former Washington *Post* feature writer and arts columnist. She has written extensively on business and economics and political affairs and has edited nonfiction books. Her recent credits include writing a script about computer literacy, and short stories, as well as the development of educational games for a children's magazine. In addition to a novel and a volume of poetry which are nearing completion, Ms. Conn is currently writing and producing a television series on the visual arts.

**Tee Corinne** is a graphic artist best known for her *Cunt Coloring Book* (a. k. a. *Labiaflowers*), *Yantras of Womanlove* (photo-erotica) and the *Sapphistry* illustrations which honor women artists who created erotica in the past. Her "Female Genitalia" slides are used in sex education classes and were published in *I Am My Lover*. Since 1977 she has designed covers for Naiad Press and in 1981 was a cofounder, with four other women, of *The Blatant Image: A Magazine of Feminist Photography*.

**Mary Beth Crain** is a freelance writer currently working as the associate entertainment editor for the *L.A. Weekly*. She has written for numerous major publications, the Los Angeles *Times*, the Chicago *Sun-Times*, the Los Angeles *Herald-Examiner*, the Detroit *Free Press*, *Playgirl*, and others. She is also the editor in chief of the *L.A. Weekly's* book *Best of L.A.*, a humorous guide to Los Angeles, and is currently working on a satiric/erotic novel based on her story "Picasso."

**Syn Ferguson** is a freelance writer and PR consultant. Her nonfiction has appeared in *Essence, Prime-Times, Reader's Digest* and others. Her poetry has been selected for presentation on the radio, and her video drama *T. Bear's Christmas* was produced for cable television. She self-publishes erotic fiction and is currently working on an erotic novel, *Evangels*.

**Susan Griffin** is the author of *Woman and Nature: The Roaring Inside Her; Pornography and Silence: Culture's Revenge Against Nature;* and *Made F(f)rom T(t)his Earth*, an anthology of her work. She has also written a play entitled *Voices*, which won an Emmy. Presently Susan is at work on a new book called *The First and Last: A Woman Who Thinks About War*.

**Signe Hammer** has published three books: *Passionate Attachments: Fathers and Daughters in America Today; Daughters and Mothers, Mothers and Daughters;* and *Women: Body and Culture: Essays on the Sexuality of Women in a Changing Society*. Her articles have appeared in publications such as *McCall's, Parade, Science Digest, Mademoiselle, Harper's Bazaar, Working Woman, Ms., Health* and *The Village Voice*. She has published prose and poetry in *Fiction* and *The New England Review* and teaches nonfiction writing at New York University.

**Robin M. Henig** is a freelance writer. She has published in the *New York Times Magazine, Woman's Day,* the Washington Post Book World, *Sci-Quest, Human Behavior* and *BioScience,* among others. She is the author of *Your Premature Baby* and *The Myth of Senility.* She has won the American Psychological Association National Media Award, the American Medical Writers Association Award for Excellence in Biomedical Writing, the American Academy of Pediatrics Journalism Award, and the National Association of Government Communicators Blue Pencil Award.

**Valerie Kelly** is a freelance writer and lives with her son. She writes advertising copy, edits magazines, creates blurbs for box covers and direct mail pieces, as well as writing erotica. She is a regular contributor to *Playgirl* and writes and edits several adult-oriented publications. So far, her novels have not been published, but she's pecking away at her fourth one anyway.

**Marian Kester** is the author of *The Dead Kennedys: An Unauthorized Biography* and *Street Art: The Punk Poster in S.F.* She is a reviewer for *S.F. Review of Books, Berkeley Graduate* and *High Performance,* to name but a few. Her essays have been published in numerous anthologies and magazines. Currently she is putting together a book comprised of thirty of her essays on men and women, sex and love, in the modern world.

**Sharon Mayes** is a psychotherapist, a teacher and a writer. In addition to various teaching positions, she has published in numerous academic journals. Her poetry has been published in *Wingspread: A Feminist Literary Journal,* and she has written two unpublished novels and is currently working on a third.

**Karen McChrystal** is a writer, journalist and therapist. She has edited and written for a number of local newspapers including the Berkeley *New Morning Newspaper* and the *City Arts Monthly,* in addition to a number of political-economic newsletters. She is currently counseling writers and working on a book on the creative process.

**Deena Metzger** is a poet, playwright, novelist and therapist. Her published books include *Skin: Shadows/Silence, The Woman Who Slept with Men to Take the War Out of Them, Tree, The Axis Mundi Poems* and *Dark Milk.* Among her plays are *Dreams Against the State, Not as Sleepwalkers* and *Book of Hags.* She has worked on video and film documentaries. In addition, poems, articles, critical pieces and other works may be found in numerous anthologies, popular and literary magazines, academic books and journals.

**Suzanne Miller** is a writer and a transformational therapist in private practice. She has published two books of poetry: *Your Fine Court Hat Before Supper and My Rain,* and *The Dark, The Light,* co-authored with her brother, E.J. Miller. One of her plays, *The Interruption,* was performed in Mill Valley under her direction. She is currently working on a novel entitled *The Autobiography of Gypsy Marlowe.*

**Lynn Scott Myers** is a fine artist and a cellist and for the past two years has held a post as proprietress of a figurative art studio-gallery called Art and Soul. She has also written a novel on aesthetics and sanity.

**Brooke Newman** is a freelance editor and writer. She was an editor at Simon and Schuster, wrote for *Manhattan East* and researched and wrote for a movie and book entitled *Sacred Grounds* and for Leon Uris in the publication of *Jerusalem.* She edited films for Stouffer Productions and was fiction editor and wrote for *Aspen Leaves.* She is presently at work on a nonfiction book as well as a novel. Most important, she is the mother of three.

**Doraine Poretz** is a poet, teacher and playwright who lives with her eleven-year-old daughter. One of her plays, *Body to Light,* has been produced in Los Angeles, and another, *The Holding,* is optioned for production in New York. Her two books of poetry are *Re: Visions* and *This Woman in America.* Her poems have been published in numerous literary magazines, and she has read her work in colleges and poetry centers throughout Los Angeles and in New York.

**Jacquie Robb** lives in Northern California with her lover and three cats. She is a writer of poetry and an occasional short story and is currently working on a novel about parthenogenesis. Meanwhile she works odd jobs to help pay the rent.

**Rayann St. Peter** is a native Texan, in her eleventh year of marriage. Longing to express the beauty around her, she has written a harvest of poetry since the age of fourteen. She had three poems published in *Writers Bloc #1,* a publication of Texas A&I University, where she is a part-time student. She is also working on a romance novel set in Hawaii.

**Dorothy Schuler** has worked for the past fifteen years in the book industry: rare and retail book sales, printing, book manufacturing and publishing. In the latter half of that period, she has been an editor, ghost writer, technical writer and book reviewer. She was senior editor at Peace Press and does freelance editing for other major publishing houses.

**Beth Tashery Shannon** has published experimental fiction in the *Pushcart Prize III* anthology and elsewhere, most recently in *Chicago Review* and *TriQuarterly*. She has also just completed an erotic first novel, *Glitter Street*, which is as yet unpublished.

**Helen A. Thomas** has been writing commentary and life-style pieces for several years. These have appeared in the Los Angeles *Herald-Examiner* and the Washington *Star-News*. She edits and writes technical material and is working on a mainstream novel about single life in Beverly Hills.

**Grace Zabriskie** is a professional actress with numerous stage, screen and television credits. She used to make a living as a silkscreen artist. She is a published poet, a screenwriter and a carpenter and lives with her husband.